Breaking the Chains of the Past

Printed in the United States of America.

ISBN: 978-1-59992-974-3

DOUGLAS DOBBERFUHL, M.S.

BREAKING THE CHAINS OF THE PAST

Overcoming Childhood Trauma Through the Power of the Atonement

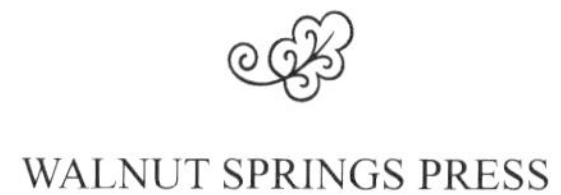

WALNUT SPRINGS PRESS

Other Books by Douglas Dobberfuhl, M.S.

Overcoming Addiction: The Journey Begins
Overcoming Addiction: A Twelve-Step Companion Guide
Healing the Codependent Heart

Table of Contents

AUTHOR'S NOTE

Throughout this book, you will read sessions based on work I did with clients. Although the sessions read like transcripts, they are actually a conglomeration of sessions, stories, and multiple clients. This prevents the disclosure of any client's true identity. In addition, all client names in this book have been changed to protect confidentiality and anonymity.

Part 1

Beginning the Journey

And it shall come to pass, that if the Gentiles shall hearken unto the Lamb of God in that day that he shall manifest himself unto them in word, and also in power, in very deed, unto the taking away of their stumbling blocks . . . —1 Nephi 14:1

Chapter 1
Finding the Miracle

From the beginning of our premortal existence, we have been taught the plan of salvation and the central role Christ would play in it. Why is He the central Figure in that plan? Because without Him, we have no chance of returning to Heavenly Father's presence and becoming perfect.

In our first estate, while we lived in the spirit world before we came to earth, we possessed moral agency. We made choices. Lucifer chose to rebel against Heavenly Father. Many of our other spirit brothers and sisters also rebelled against the Father's plan. As Brent L. Top explained, "The war in heaven involved much more than just voting for plans of salvation. It undoubtedly involved a war of words, a war for the hearts, minds, souls and strength of all of God's children" (Top, 1988).

Here on earth, in our second estate, we still have agency and the ability to make choices. When our choices go against the teachings of Heavenly Father, those choices often hurt others. In fact, rarely can we break one of the Lord's commandments without that choice hurting someone else. Sin does not exist in a vacuum, meaning there is no such thing as a victimless sin. Elder Quentin L. Cook of the Quorum of the Twelve Apostles stated: "Some challenges result from the agency of others. Agency is essential for individual spiritual growth and development. Evil conduct is an element of agency. Captain Moroni explained this very important doctrine: 'The Lord suffereth the righteous to be slain that his justice and judgment may come upon the wicked.' He made it clear that the righteous are not lost but 'enter into the rest of the Lord their God' (Alma 60:13). The wicked will be held accountable for the atrocities they perpetrate" (Cook, 2011).

The Savior's sacrifice would not only allow us to repent of sinful choices, but would allow both offender and victim to be healed if they so desired. We can enter into the Lord's rest here and now. We can find peace here and now. But if one chooses not to repent of past abusive and evil acts, then just as in the first estate, there will come a time when choices made here will demand a full and final recompense.

By virtue of temple work for the dead, we know repentance continues in our next estate. Overcoming sin and healing from past traumas will continue until the Final Judgment. At every stage of the Father's plan, the Savior's Atonement is essential. Therefore, it is vital that we understand how to access its marvelous power.

Wade, a client of mine, recounted in a frustrated tone how he had become very disillusioned with the Atonement. He said he hated it when people got up and bore their testimonies about how the Atonement saved them, helped them, or healed them. He waited to hear *how* it happened, but no one ever explained that. For Wade, the Atonement had become an unsolvable puzzle. He knew the Atonement bore fruit in many people's lives, yet he remained on the outside, feeling confused and perplexed. It wasn't that he didn't feel the Spirit testify of the reality of the Atonement. In fact, that frustrated him even more. He understood that he could be forgiven through the Atonement, but he couldn't find concrete ways to utilize its power in all areas of his life.

Wade is not alone with his thoughts. As I sit across from members of the Church struggling in therapy, I routinely hear these types of comments:

- "My bishop told me to let the Savior heal me, but I don't know how to do that."
- "I believe the Atonement helps people repent, but I have no idea how it can help me overcome my childhood abuse."
- "I don't know how to do it—I don't know how to connect to the Atonement."

Like Wade, you have no doubt heard countless talks and testimonies in sacrament meeting where the person mentions how wonderful the Atonement is, how powerful it is, and how life-changing it can be. Yet the practical application—the nuts and bolts of how to gain access to the Atonement—often feels elusive. How frustrating it is to be members of Christ's Church and not know how to use the most precious gift He has given us—His great and everlasting sacrifice.

As an author, therapist, and fellow traveler of this difficult journey of healing and recovery, I have asked my own questions about how to make the leap from seeing the vastness of the Atonement to having an intimate, personal experience with it. I toyed with the idea of writing about this subject for several years, but was never inspired. It wasn't until I did the hard work of actually doing what I wanted to write about that ideas started to flow.

The aim of this book is to help survivors of childhood abuse—whether it be emotional, physical, or sexual—in two ways. The first is to help readers understand the stumbling blocks that come from childhood trauma that keep us from embracing the power of the Atonement. The second is to explore concrete, how-to methods of applying and gaining the promised healing that Christ offers us.

One of the biggest stumbling blocks is that of our pain and the need for justice. Thoughts of how unfair the past has been can eat away at our insides until we are only a bitter, empty husk of a person. We seek for justice and vengeance. We want to make our offenders take responsibility for what they did, but this rarely occurs. Somebody has to pay, we cry out, but the reality is, it is we who have to pay the bill. Those who gave us this pain cannot take it back. These wounds are ours now. Even if our abusers do apologize, nothing they do can erase the pain. We must pay the price to find healing and resolution. Elder Richard G Scott spoke about this need for justice and how it can derail healing. "Rest assured that the Perfect Judge, Jesus the Christ, with a perfect knowledge of the details, will hold all abusers accountable for every unrighteous act. In time He will fully apply the required demands of justice unless there is complete repentance. *Your preoccupation with a need for justice only slows your healing and allows the perpetrator to continue his abusive control*" (Scott, 2008; italics added).

As always, however, the Atonement offers us hope. In the aforementioned conference talk from Elder Quentin L Cook, he spoke about trials and the harsh unfairness that life offers us. "Regardless of the trials we face in this life, the Savior's Atonement provides lifeboats for everyone. For those who think the trials they face are unfair, the Atonement covers all of the unfairness of life" (Cook, 2011). It is interesting to note that Elder Cook repeats this statement in various ways at least two more times. Toward the end of the discourse, he testifies that "Jesus Christ . . . is our Savior and Redeemer, whose Atonement not only provides for salvation and exaltation but also will compensate for all the unfairness of life" (ibid).

No one understands the sense of being stuck, trapped, and defeated more than the Savior. He understands our desire for justice. He understands how utterly unfair life can be. He knows intimately the horrible pain that cripples us emotionally, spiritually, and even sometimes physically. No matter how dark, how hopeless, or how alone we feel, I testify that healing is possible. Burdens are lifted. Enormous shifts in beliefs and perspectives happen a little here and a little there. Freedom can be achieved.

Sometimes we feel as though we have been slugging away in the mud and the muck for weeks, months, or even years, seeing very little progress. And then there are these moments that defy description. We are plucked up out of the mire and taken to a mountain. There we see the majesty and beauty of a sunrise or a sunset. We can see so much more than the smelly swamplands of our past. We can breathe. We can stretch out and not feel confined, closed in, or crushed by the fear and terror of our past.

Over time, we have more and more of these moments. Then comes the moment where we realize we don't have to go back anymore. We are struck with awe and a profound sense of wonder. How is it done? The answer is and always has been (even if we didn't know it, or always feel it) Jesus Christ and His loving, patient, outstretched arms.

He is not a God who sits far away. He is in the trenches with us, cheering us on, motivating us (sometimes with what can feel like a two-by-four), encouraging us, crying with us, hugging us, and celebrating with us. There is not one tear I have shed along this journey that was not matched by my Elder Brother Jesus Christ. Sometimes, His lap was my pillow as I struggled for a moment's peace. Sometimes He reached inside and dislodged some dark emotional sludge to help me breathe easier. Sometimes He hugged me and filled me with incredible light and love. I am free because of my Savior. I am saved from the destructiveness and total darkness of my past because of Him. He is my everything—Master, Counselor, Confidant, Healer, and Father of my rebirth.

Let's go find Him together.

CHAPTER 2
SESSION WITH TERRI

"I don't want to pray," Terri said with a bit of defiance in her voice.

"Why not?" I asked.

"Because God doesn't want to hear from me."

"Because . . ."

"Because I'm sure He thinks I'm terrible."

"Why would He think that?"

"Because I *am* terrible!"

"Are you terrible because of the abuse?"

"Yes. I'm disgusting. I'm bad. I'm garbage."

"The abuse wasn't your fault. You were a child."

"Doesn't matter. It's infected me. Now not even God wants me."

"How do you know that?"

"Because I don't even want me!" she yelled, smashing her balled-up fists into the couch. Somehow, admitting that unlocked something inside of Terri and she burst into tears. I sat watching, saying nothing. She sobbed and repeated the statement over and over: "I don't even want me."

After a few moments, she reached for a tissue and blew her nose. During this pause, I said, "So you believe that God thinks the same way you do about yourself—that how He sees you and thinks about you is based on how you think and feel about yourself?"

Terri nodded slightly.

"Did you feel this way before you were abused?"

She paused for a moment. "I don't remember before I was abused."

"How did you feel when you got baptized?"

Terri took another tissue and tried to wipe off the mascara running down her cheeks. "I hoped that all the bad things that happened to me would be washed away and I would feel clean."

"And did you?"

"No."

"Did you feel anything?"

Terri thought for a moment and then nodded her head. "Yeah, I felt hopeful."

"Hopeful about what?"

"That maybe God really was there and that He was going to help me."

"Did He?"

"Two weeks after I was baptized, the neighbor sexually abused me. So no, God did not help me. And from that moment on, I knew nothing could make me clean and that God didn't help me because I was dirty. His baptism wasn't powerful enough to make me clean and acceptable."

I leaned forward and said as earnestly as I could, "Terri, the dirtiness that you feel isn't yours. The infection you talk about didn't come from you, and it isn't yours. This stuff inside you was put there by very bad people—"

"Doesn't matter," she interrupted.

"Yes, it does. If you had a beautiful white blanket and the dog came in from outside and walked on it, leaving dirty paw prints on it, would you throw it out?"

"If I couldn't get it clean."

"What if you had special detergent—really strong detergent—that could get your dirty blanket gleaming white again?"

"Then I suppose I'd wash it," Terri said grudgingly.

"Right! And all that dirt would be gone. It is the same with you. You aren't responsible for that dirt getting there. Someone else left it there. And through the Savior's Atonement, that dirt can be taken away and you can become clean and whole."

Terri rolled her eyes. "You sound just like the bishop. He's always talking about how I need the Savior in my life, how I need more faith, how I just need to pray more." She shook her head in anger. "What does he know? Was he ever raped at age four when he went camping with his uncle? Or was he kidnapped and sexually assaulted by a pedophile who worked as a clown? Huh? No!"

She raised her hands in the air, exasperated. "Of course I have prayed. I have gone to the temple. I have gotten priesthood blessings. I have read my scriptures. And none of it works! The bishop has no idea what will help. I bet he gives the same answers to everyone that comes to see him."

"It must be pretty demoralizing to turn to spiritual practices, hoping for something to change, and then nothing does," I said quietly.

"It is. Now do you understand why I know that God doesn't want me?"

I nodded. "Yeah, I understand why you think that."

"I don't think it—I know it!" Terri growled.

I shrugged my shoulders. "So what are you going to do? It looks like you're stuck. God doesn't want you. You don't want you. You are broken and dirty and infected. You lost, they won. They beat you and you stayed down."

Terri nodded. "Yes, now you finally get it. I am hopeless. I am beyond help."

"Okay. So are you going to lie down and die? Have you written a goodbye letter to your husband and kids?"

"What? I'm not going to kill myself!" Terri said indignantly.

"But I thought you said it was all over."

"It is, but—"

"So why are you here in therapy, Terri, if it's over?" I interrupted her. "People usually come to counseling because at the very least they want to believe there is hope for things to change."

"Stop twisting things!"

"Oh, I see. You just came here to get me to understand how bad you are."

"Yes!" she exclaimed almost triumphantly.

"And then what?" I asked.

Terri looked confused. "What do you mean?"

"Well, I do understand. I do see. You are a worthless piece of garbage. So now what?"

"You aren't going to try to save me?"

I shook my head. "Nope. Can't change something that doesn't want to be changed."

"Can't. Can't be changed," she corrected me.

"Right, can't be changed," I echoed. "You want to change, but you can't."

Terri looked confused again. "Yeah, I guess that's right."

"You would like to feel clean and whole and loved again, but it will never happen."

"Uh-huh."

"You would like to have the chains of your abusive past broken. You would like to be free. You would like to feel alive again, but you know those things can never happen."

Terri's expression softened. The anger, the bitterness, the self-hatred slipped away. She didn't even respond, just gave a slight nod.

I pushed a little more. "You would like to feel nurtured, safe, and secure. You would love for someone to really listen to you and validate your experiences. You would love for Heavenly Father to come down and wrap His arms around you and hold you tight. But that can never be, right?"

There was silence. I barely breathed and let the silence just be. I could hear the clock ticking on the wall. Terri was looking down, not saying anything. She appeared almost frozen. I waited, sensing that something was happening inside of her. I prayed silently.

Finally she looked up, tears welling in her eyes, and with a very soft, trembling voice asked the question I had been praying she would ask. "Could it really be?"

I gave a slight smile and nodded. Now we could start working.

Chapter 3
The Reality of the Problem

I sat in a room with a client, Jennifer, plus her husband and parents. Jennifer trembled slightly. Over the past several weeks, I had asked her repeatedly if she was sure she wanted to do this. Her parents were actually her biological aunt and uncle, who had adopted Jennifer after her mother gave up her parental rights due to her chronic drug use. Jennifer's aunt felt angry and resentful that she had to take her sister's child. When Jennifer was with her aunt and uncle, now her legal parents, she often felt put down. Yet she was certain this was the course of action she wanted to take.

As we got started, Jennifer said, "Mom and Dad, when I was little, I was abused by Glenn and Sarah." Glenn and Sarah were her aunt and uncle's older children, raised as her siblings. Her aunt gasped and her uncle's face became even more stoic. Jennifer continued, "It's why I spent so much time outside when I was little. If I was outside, I was safe from them. I have been keeping this a secret for years." As the primary breadwinner, the aunt was often out of the house. The uncle picked up work where he could, often traveling out of state for jobs. This left Jennifer alone with her older cousins, unsupervised, for great lengths of time.

The meeting went surprisingly well. Jennifer's aunt hugged her, cried, and apologized for being distant and cold. Her uncle reminded her how much they loved her. In some ways this was an end to nearly a year and a half of counseling. In other ways, it was the beginning of creating a new and healthy connection to her family.

Jennifer is one of many whose lives have been affected by abuse. The numbers are shocking. According to the National Sexual Violence Resource Center, one in four girls and one in six boys are sexually abused before their eighteenth birthdays (NSVRC, 2012).

ChildHelp, one of the largest national non-profit organizations dedicated to preventing and treating child abuse, routinely produces a document outlining the level of abuse occurring in the United States. The following statistics come from one of ChildHelp's recent publications:

- A report of child abuse is made every ten seconds.
- More than four children die every day as a result of child abuse.
- More than 90% of juvenile sexual abuse victims know their perpetrator.
- Child abuse occurs at every socioeconomic level, across ethnic and cultural lines, within all religions, and at all levels of education.
- About 30% of abused and neglected children will later abuse their own children, continuing the cycle of abuse.
- In at least one study, about 80% of twenty-one-year-olds who were abused as children met criteria for at least one psychological disorder.
- Of all the reported, investigated, and founded cases of child abuse in 2009 in the United States, 20% of the abuse was physical and 10% was sexual. Emotional abuse was so prevalent in all the various categories, it was not measured. (ChildHelp, 2013)

Childhood trauma encompasses more than physical, sexual, and emotional abuse. Neglect, poverty, hunger, chronic pain and illness, divorce, peer rejection (bullying, name calling, teasing), and even marital discord impact children in deep and profound ways.

Prophets have always counseled God's children to love others and treat them with respect. The last five Presidents of The Church of Jesus Christ of Latter Day Saints have specifically declared that abuse in any form is absolutely unacceptable.

President Spencer W. Kimball

There are not enough good homes. Children still come to some homes where they will be abused, not loved, and not taught the truth. We are greatly concerned with the fact that the press continues to report many cases of child abuse. We are much concerned that there would be a single parent that would inflict damages on a child. The Lord loved little children, and he said: "Suffer little children, and forbid them not, to come unto me: for of such is the kingdom of heaven." (Matt. 19:14.) Let no Latter-day Saint parent ever be guilty of the heinous crime of abusing one of Christ's little ones! (Kimball, 1978)

Ezra Taft Benson

This title [of my talk] is prompted by reports that have recently come to my attention about the shocking actions of some fathers and husbands, and their unrighteous actions involve wife and child abuse. As I have listened to these reports, I have asked myself, "How can any member of the Church—any man who holds the priesthood of God—be guilty of cruelty to his own wife and children? Such actions, if practiced by a priesthood holder, are almost inconceivable. They are totally out of character with the teachings of the Church and the gospel of Jesus Christ. (Benson, 1983)

President Howard W. Hunter

You who hold the priesthood must not be abusive in your relationship with children. Seek always to employ the principles of priesthood government set forth in the revelations (see D&C 93:40; D&C 121:34–36, 41–45). President George Albert Smith wisely counseled: "We should not lose our tempers and abuse one another. . . . Nobody ever abused anybody else when he had the spirit of the Lord. It is always when we have some other spirit" (in Conference Report, Oct. 1950, p. 8). No man who has been ordained to the priesthood of God can with impunity abuse his wife or child. Sexual abuse of children has long been a cause for excommunication from the Church. (Hunter, 1994)

President Gordon B. Hinckley

Then there is the terrible, inexcusable, and evil phenomenon of physical and sexual abuse. It is unnecessary. It is unjustified. It is indefensible. In terms of physical abuse, I have never accepted the principle of "spare the rod and spoil the child." . . . I am persuaded that violent fathers produce violent sons. I am satisfied that such punishment in most instances does more damage than good. Children don't need beating. They need love and encouragement. They need fathers to whom they can look with respect rather than fear. Above all, they need example.

And then there is the terrible, vicious practice of sexual abuse. It is beyond understanding. It is an affront to the decency that ought to exist in every man and woman. It is a violation of that which is sacred and divine. It is destructive in the lives of children. It is reprehensible and worthy of the most severe condemnation. Shame on any man or woman who would sexually abuse a child. In doing so, the abuser not only does the most serious kind of injury. He or she also stands condemned before the Lord.

It was the Master himself who said, "But whoso shall offend one of these little ones which believe in me, it were better for him that a millstone were hanged about his neck, and that he were drowned in the depth of the sea" (Matt. 18:6). How could he have spoken in stronger terms? (Hinckley, 1994)

President Thomas S. Monson

If only all children had loving parents, safe homes, and caring friends, what a wonderful world would be theirs. Unfortunately, not all children are so bounteously blessed. Some children witness their fathers savagely beating their mothers, while others are on the receiving end of such abuse. What cowardice, what depravity, what shame!

Local hospitals everywhere receive these little ones, bruised and battered, accompanied by bald-faced lies that the child "ran into the door" or "fell down the stairs." Liars, bullies who abuse children, they will one day reap the whirlwind of their foul deeds. The quiet, the hurt, the offended child victim of abuse, and at times incest, must receive help.

A district judge, in a letter to me, declared, "Sexual abuse of children is one of the most depraved, destructive, and demoralizing crimes in civilized society. There is an alarming increase of reported physical, psychological, and sexual abuse of children. Our courts are becoming inundated with this repulsive behavior.

The Church does not condone such heinous and vile conduct. Rather, we condemn in the harshest of terms such treatment of God's precious children. Let the child be rescued, nurtured, loved, and healed. Let the offender be brought to justice, to accountability, for his actions and receive professional treatment to curtail such wicked and devilish conduct. When you and I know of such conduct and fail to take action to eradicate it, we become part of the problem. We share part of the guilt. We experience part of the punishment. (Monson, 1991)

Spanning nearly fifty years, these prophets make it very plain that abuse is not and will not be tolerated by Church leaders. That they need to speak about this to members of the Lord's true Church shows that childhood abuse is present everywhere. Being a member of the Church does not exempt anyone from the ravages of evil.

Clearly, the reality of childhood abuse is known to God and His servants. With outstretched arms, they invite all who have been burdened by abuse to come unto Christ and be healed. The process may be slow, but every step toward experiencing the Savior's balm of soothing comfort is worth it.

Just as real as abuse is, so also is the reality of the cure. Let's discover it together.

Chapter 4
Trauma and the Brain

Out of all the major systems within the human body, the brain is the most adaptive, flexible, and malleable. It constantly reacts to the external environment—to positive as well as negative experiences. When a child is abused, the brain is affected in a myriad of ways. For an individual who has been abused, these brain alterations can be a major stumbling block in accessing the Atonement. Trauma's profound impact on the brain often makes it difficult for the person to experience the healing power of the Savior's love.

To some degree, abuse affects all aspects of a child's life. Like a computer virus, trauma can seep into all major functions of the child's body, causing a total and systemic alteration. The human body is sensitive to abuse, and emotional and mental wounds can have a significant impact on the way the body operates. The good news is that just as the brain can adapt as a result of enduring trauma, it can also change as a result of experiencing healing and recovery. For every negative consequence, there will be hope as well. If abuse can mold a brain to operate a certain way, God can reshape the brain to overcome the effects of that abuse.

Normally, if an individual is without birth defects and grows up in a healthy, functional environment, the brain will become an integrated, functional organ. A functional brain has the chemicals necessary to enable full communication with all of its various parts. However, the brain of a child raised in a dysfunctional, traumatic, or abusive environment often shows harmful effects. Various parts of the brain will have difficulty sharing information, and naturally occurring chemicals may be underproduced or overproduced, causing errors in thinking or feeling.

When these things occur, the body can enter a state of adaptation built around survival. This adaptation may be beneficial when it occurs, but if left unchecked, it usually causes problems later by inhibiting personal growth and the ability to learn healthy coping mechanisms. As Linda Graham stated, "Unless new experiences cause a rewiring of the old circuits, the patterns of coping we learn as toddlers become our default responses to life's perils and pitfalls" (Graham, 2013). If our experiences as toddlers were less than healthy, we will create coping strategies that are either unstable and chaotic or rigid and inflexible.

World-renowned researcher Bessel van der Kolk explains that individuals who experience trauma and are diagnosed with post-traumatic stress disorder (PTSD) exhibit disturbances in neurotransmitters—specifically, dopamine, serotonin, and norepinephrine. The depletion of and disturbances in these neurotransmitters leave the abused individual feeling unbalanced (van der Kolk, 1994).

This unbalance sets the stage for the individual to seek ways to feel better—or at the very least, to not feel the discomfort that comes with abuse. Often the person finds his or her own "balance" with substances such as alcohol and illegal drugs. Such use frequently leads to addiction (Dapice, Inkanish, & Brauchi, 2001).

Before long, these maladaptive behaviors become a way to self-medicate and self-regulate because they temporarily ease the individual out of depression and anxiety. The behaviors also bring release from pain and fear, at least momentarily. Sometimes the acting-out behaviors bring a rush that lasts for days. Indeed, the more an individual acts out in his or her addiction, the more the brain will release soothing, intoxicating hormones and endorphins.

Someone who experiences high levels of stress (such as abuse), or even someone who experiences a lower level of constant stress (being raised in a chaotic, dysfunctional home) can have his or her brain chemicals negatively impacted. One example is the chemical monoamine oxidase (MAO). Excessive MAO production can create too much norepinephrine, which depletes serotonin. This depletion, in turn, causes the person to experience high levels of anxiety, feelings of tension and depression, and sleep disturbances. If the MAO enzymes are depleted through overuse, then serotonin, dopamine, and norepinephrine can be overproduced. All of these chemical surpluses can cause hyperactivity, exaggerated sexuality, the rapid change of ideas, and decreased sleep.

Individuals with attachment problems due to childhood abuse and trauma can also have decreased levels of oxytocin and vasopressin, which can cause relationship problems in the future. Dr. Rebecca Turner and Dr. Teresa McGuinness conducted a study on the impact of stress on oxytocin. They discovered that stress and negative experiences lower oxytocin levels. Then, as oxytocin levels dropped, study participants reported feeling anxiety in their close relationships (Turner and McGuinness, 1999). Indeed, abnormalities (deficiencies) in the neural pathways for either oxytocin or vasopressin can often enhance repetitive behaviors and can negatively impact social learning and the ability to emotionally connect to other people (Hollander et al, 2003).

Trauma and Brain Regions

The brain is highly sensitive to abuse and trauma. Numerous studies have revealed the connection between trauma and brain function. Let's explore some areas of the brain and review studies that prove what childhood trauma can do to it.

Left Temporal Lobe

Jay Goldstein states that children who have experienced psychological, physical, and/or sexual abuse tend to have abnormalities in the left temporal lobe—the area of the brain that deals with memory and emotion. This makes it difficult to effectively handle emotions. Indeed, people diagnosed with posttraumatic stress disorder often lose the capacity to use emotional states as a way to navigate and connect with the outside world. Instead of using feelings as cues to attend to incoming information, arousal of anxiety occurs in its place, kicking in the flight-or-fight response (Goldstein, 2001). Van der Kolk offers added insight to what this looks like for traumatized individuals: "Hence, they are prone to go immediately from stimulus to response without making the necessary psychological assessment of the meaning of what is going on. This makes them prone to freeze, or alternatively, to overreact and intimidate others in response to minor provocations" (van der Kolk, 1994).

Medial Prefrontal Cortex

Another part of the brain affected by abuse is the medial prefrontal cortex. As this area changes according to the impact of trauma, the individual struggles with "pathological emotional responses" (Bremner, 2000). Simply put, the victim will respond to a certain variable from the abuse even if the abuse is not currently happening, like being afraid of dark places even if now there is nothing to fear in the dark, or having a strong negative reaction from seeing or feeling pubic hair even if the person has grown up and is now in an adult relationship. In other words, some aspect of the trauma gets stuck and triggers a negative reaction—usually fear or disgust—years after the event happened.

Corpus Callosum

According to Joan Arehart-Treichel, "It appears as if the psychological impact of childhood abuse can damage the corpus callosum—the major information pathway between the two brain hemispheres" (Arehart-Treichel, 2001). In one of their studies, Treichel and her associates found that sexual abuse in girls was associated with a major reduction in the size of the corpus callosum (ibid). This explains why information about a particular experience can be stored in a fragmented manner, and why integration and communication with major areas of the brain can be hampered.

Limbic System

As a person experiences trauma, another part of the brain is impacted, namely the limbic system, which governs mood. "The psychological impact ensuing from childhood physical abuse appears capable of damaging the cerebellar vermis, an area of the brain involved in emotion, attention, and the regulation of the limbic system" (ibid). The ability to regulate mood and affect (how we handle emotions) become impaired due to trauma, often either causing the individual to be constricted in handling his or her emotions (narrowing them or squeezing them out of existence), or to be very labile (have all-over-the-place feelings). This affects the relaxation or constriction of the organs of our body. It is mood, not thought, that affects the physical health of our internal organs. Innumerable studies have proven that the chemicals that run the body and the brain are the same chemicals that involve emotion. As Elaine de Beauport explains, "To restrict feeling is to restrict the organs of our body and leads to eventual weakness" (Dayton, 2001).

Mark Schwartz, a noted author and therapist, talks about how often the affect—the emotional memories of past abuse—leak into the adult's life, while the cognitive memory remains missing.

Enactment occurs instead of remembering. What this means is that a person can have vivid emotional memories spring up about the abuse, but that's it—just a sudden overflow of intense emotion. The facts, or snapshots of the abuse, remain locked in the brain. So instead of actually remembering the abuse, the emotional explosion feels as if the person is actually re-enacting the abuse. Often this comes in the form of a flashback.

Hippocampus

Another major part of the brain that is affected by PTSD is the hippocampus, which will shrink in size as a result of trauma. This will affect memory—specifically, the ability to recall trauma—and make it difficult to learn new things. This new information helps to understand delayed or recovered memories of abuse. Many times an adult who had no previous memory of suffering from childhood abuse will suddenly be inundated with "new" or recovered memories. Although it has sparked great controversy within the therapeutic community, the ongoing research on the hippocampus has given critical evidence to support this phenomenon.

The Brain and Spirituality

Biological evidence supports the idea that as humans, we are wired, designed, and created to be spiritual. Therefore, anything that decreases or quells our innate spirituality will cause problems in our lives. Summarized from Danah Zohar and Dr. Ian Marshall's book *Spiritual Intelligence: The Ultimate Intelligence,* the new brain research provides the following revolutionary information on our hard-wired spirituality:

- There is no physical neural connection linking all the neurons in the brain. The brain consists of many independent "expert systems." Yet there is a "higher order" system connecting these systems together, allowing them to communicate with each other. It acts as a unifier. This system is the synchronous neural oscillations in the 40 Hz range. All neurons oscillate (vibrate) when stimulated. Without this special brain wave, our world would consist of meaningless fragments. Unless we integrate our spiritual experiences into our consciousness, these connections with Heaven will have very little impact on us.

- This oscillation—brain wave vibration—is the brain's neural process devoted to unifying and giving meaning to our experience, a neural process that literally "binds" our experiences together. It brings together and connects the rational-thought-processes part of the brain with the emotional-driven, pattern-recognizing, habit-building parts of the brain to create a unifying "wholeness" to the brain.
- When this form of communicating occurs, it allows us to be creative, flexible, visionary, and spontaneous. This system enables us to have a deep sense of what life's struggles are about. "The brain, in short, was *designed* to be conscious, and *designed* to have a transcendent dimension" (Zohar and Marshall, 2000, 76).
- When a person experiences trauma, a splitting or separation occurs, both physically and psychologically. The brain (as well as the body) begins to compartmentalize these experiences as a way to survive. Therefore, it can be difficult to understand, grasp, integrate, and put into proper context the trauma experienced. Parts of the self become blocked from communicating with other parts. Denial, repression, trying to normalize the trauma, minimizing, blocking, numbing—all are the consequences of the disruption of the brain wave unifier. Zohar and Marshall call this state "wounded fragmentation" (ibid, 9).

This woundedness affects one's ability to sense, understand, and grasp meaning in life. Being cut off, the individual's thought processes and emotional responses and regulation become limited and fragmented. Behavioral symptoms and psychological problems erupt, such as depression, obsessions, mania, narcissism, self-loathing, self-indulgence, and grandiosity. Addictions often grow out of this "troubled garden."

The biological evidence just mentioned shows that a spiritually healthy person is one who is whole, integrated, and honest with his or her past and present. Continuing to use our trauma-based coping skills to handle regular life keeps us spiritually stunted and unaware of ourselves. Therefore, healing and recovery is necessary to regain wholeness, decrease that chronic compartmentalization and disconnection, and restore balance and meaning to our lives.

The good news is that the brain can heal. The brain and body can be reconnected. It is absolutely possible to restore the communication within our bodies that promotes and creates wholeness and integration.

As this occurs, our intimate connection with Heavenly Father begins to mean something. Countless people with traumatic pasts claim to be religious and spiritual, yet still struggle to heal from their pasts. Why? In part, because they have yet to find *meaning* in their relationship with God. Unless we work on becoming aware and integrating our past with our present, our relationship with God will simply be the letters G-O-D. It will not hold the meaning that sparks and creates significant change.

Let's find those sparks. Let's discover our stories and allow Christ to write the next few pages in the book of our lives.

Chapter 5
Why We Need Help

In 1999, the ACL ligament in my left knee ripped in half. I thought I had broken my leg. The pain was so shockingly intense I nearly passed out. After a few moments, I seemed to detach from the pain. I hobbled to my car and drove myself to see the doctor. They were surprised I could do this, especially since I drove a stick shift. By this time my knee was so swollen I couldn't bend it even if I wanted to. After identifying the problem, doctors scheduled surgery.

About a month and a half passed between the injury and the surgery to repair it. During that time I learned to walk with a brace, then with crutches, and then limp around without any help. I almost wondered if I needed the surgery. After all, I could drive, I had learned how to slide up and down stairs, and I could limp well enough around.

After the surgery, my left leg was put into a machine that automatically bent my knee every few minutes. The doctor wanted to make sure scar tissue didn't form in the wound and disable my knee. A few days later, I went to see the physical therapist, John. He happened to be my next-door neighbor, which worked out well because I was hesitant to do anything with my left leg. I went to therapy two to three times a week.

One day John took me out into the hall without my crutches and told me he was going to teach me how to walk again.

I laughed at him and said, "I think I know how to walk."

"Okay, show me," he replied. He folded his arms and leaned against the hospital wall. I laughed nervously and asked for my crutches. "Nope, no crutches."

"But what about my knee?"

"Your knee is strong enough." He shooed me away with his hand. "Go on—go walk."

I stood there in the hallway and reminded myself that I had been walking for nearly thirty years, so this was no big deal. Then why was I sweating? Why did I feel tense and scared? I took a step with my right leg, but could barely make my left leg move.

Suddenly John was by my side, holding me up. "Why can't I walk?" I asked, shocked at my utter failure.

"Because your brain believes your left leg isn't working. It still believes it's broken and that you need to stay off it. We have to prove to your brain that the ACL ligament is fixed and healed enough for you to walk."

"You mean it's stuck in the trauma of the past," I said, thinking out loud.

John smiled. "You just can't turn off your counseling brain, can you?" he teased me.

For the next two weeks, he taught me how to walk again. We took everything apart—from how the heel hits the floor, to what the toes do to help balance and push the foot off the ground, to what the calf muscles do, to how my knee bends. Through it all, something inside of me was confused. Part of me had memory of how to walk, and part of me was terrified of walking. John kept telling me this was more about retraining my mind and body than about teaching me something new.

Then the day came where he took me to the hospital stairwell. "We're going to go up the stairs," he declared.

My heart started thumping in my chest. I gave him a nervous look and asked, "Are you sure I am ready?"

John nodded. "We'll take it one step at a time." Instead of letting me do my usual hop-twist-shuffle, he taught me the mechanics of lifting one leg, putting pressure on it, and then using the planted leg to lift the other one. I was amazed at how unsure I was. A voice inside my head kept saying my knee wasn't strong enough and that I'd hurt it all over again. I was afraid of feeling that sharp, intense pain again.

But since I trusted John, I took a deep breath, and (even though my brain was telling me not to) started to climb up the stairs. It amazed me to see how many different parts of my body were used in going up and down stairs. John constantly corrected me so I would unlearn all the maladaptive ways I had taught myself to go up and down the stairs with my hurt knee. Eventually I was walking and going up and down stairs without having to visualize what I needed to do next and take it step by step. I just did it.

A couple of years went by. One day as I was standing in the kitchen, my wife stood back and studied me for a moment. "Why are you leaning to the right?" she asked. I didn't realize it, but I was. Whenever I stood, I would favor my left leg and lean a little heavier on my right. I did it when I shaved, standing in front of the bathroom mirror. I did it when I was cooking in the kitchen. I did it when I was standing and talking to people in the foyer at church. I was always slightly leaning.

So back to physical therapy I went. I was living in a new city and didn't have John to rely on. But the new therapist was nice and totally understood what was happening. My brain still believed my new ACL ligament wasn't strong enough to hold me up. The therapist introduced me to a whole new set of exercises. Some involved hopping, some were lunges, and some were as simple as jogging in place. The more intricate ones, where I had to completely rely on my knees, filled me with anxiety—much like walking without my crutches for the first time.

Today I don't lean. I can run, walk, and ride a bike. However, even though it has been fifteen years since the surgery, on days where I do too much sitting, my knee will begin to click. It's a sign that scar tissue is building up and I need to get out there and move around.

I tell this story to show how childhood trauma is a lot like healing from my knee injury. Left to myself, I discovered all sorts of ways to move around. In the minute-by-minute short term, these adaptive techniques helped me to remain mobile. Just like dealing with my injury, many children are left to themselves with their abuse. Traumatized children will employ many adaptive and creative strategies to manage their abusive experiences.

In the long term, my adaptive techniques to work around my severed ACL ligament actually created stumbling blocks for future healing. My little twists and turns became maladaptive, making it harder for me to adopt healthy ways to move. I had to fight against them and learn new ways to move that would ensure total freedom for my left knee.

Similarly, for adult survivors of childhood abuse, over time the short-term adaptive strategies to manage trauma become maladaptive problems. These problems inhibit the survivors' ability to overcome and heal from the abuse. And even when these strategies are identified, it takes time to replace them.

Just as my wife noticed my leaning years after the surgery, some coping strategies of adult survivors of abuse take time to discover, even after years of therapy. Many individuals' recovery and healing from childhood issues is like peeling away layers of an onion. As one layer is exposed and worked through, there seems to be another that is waiting to be discovered.

And even after everything is said and done, I still need to stay active or my knee will fill up with scar tissue and all that work and effort and pain will be for nothing. Likewise, adult survivors of childhood abuse need to focus attention on maintaining healthy ways to handle relationships and emotions. Spirituality and maintaining a close connection to God will need to be an ongoing daily goal, even if the individual no longer requires counseling.

The following is a list of maladaptive strategies that need to be addressed and removed/replaced. It is not an all-inclusive list. There may be issues you are struggling with that aren't mentioned. These are simply some of the most common symptoms of maladaptive reactions to childhood trauma. These become the stumbling blocks to accessing the Atonement of Jesus Christ.

- Getting stuck on justice or revenge, holding resentments, feeling rage or blind fury
- Perfectionism; unrealistic expectations; finding fault; being aggressive, critical, or rigid; lack of empathy for self
- Addictions; taking risks; being impulsive, self-destructive, or ignorant to consequences
- Codependency, people pleasing, acting the martyr, overcompensating, being needless and wantless
- Sleep problems
- Eating disorders
- Owning the abuse—feeling it is your fault
- Dissociating, numbness, paralysis, memory problems
- Blocking emotions, disconnection between mind and body, overly intellectual
- Anxiety, panic attacks, hypervigilance, always in heightened state of threat, overreacting
- Depression, despondency, despair
- Being passive, lack of taking ownership for life, feeling self-pity
- Isolation

- Self-harm
- Lack of discretion or discernment, boundary problems
- Self-hatred—seeing self as inadequate, unlovable, worthless
- Lack of self-care
- Loss of trust in self
- Suicidal tendency

Ironically, the more we try to distance ourselves from the past, the more our past demands to be seen, heard, and acknowledged. As Stephen Wolinski, founder of Quantum Psychology states, "An experience once resisted persists until the person is willing to 'experience the experience'" (Wolinksi, 1991). We cannot escape our past. We are not meant to. We are created and wired to connect to the daily events in our lives, regardless of how terrible they may be.

The first step in healing helps us see that we can't escape the abuse of our past. It helps to recognize that every manner or form of escape from the truth is actually making life more unmanageable. At some point, in some way, the truth of our experiences will not be contained and will demand to be spoken. There is too much energy behind truth. Maybe that's why secrets are so damaging to those that keep them.

Creating some rudimentary connection to our childhood abuse can leave us feeling wrung out, shell-shocked, and deeply troubled. For me, it was as if I was experiencing the past abuse without any shield or filter or protection. It was raw and visceral. When I went to counseling, I was a wreck for two or three days after. I was short tempered, withdrawn, and nervous. Sometimes I slept a lot. Other times I would pace, filled with an electric energy that kept me wired for hours.

I came to see my emotional, mental, and spiritual wounds as if they were infected. I would describe them in therapy like they were rotting meat, with maggots scurrying over the pungent, greenish-yellow wound. The wounds seemed so big; they touched every aspect of my life. It was a total and complete invasion. Seeing the damage and recognizing the ripple effects the abuse caused in my life filled me with despair. And for a time, meaning a few years, therapy was a small comfort. Counseling was not as much about creating peace as it was about draining the infected wounds, scraping away the rot, and cleaning out the gaping holes in my soul. Only after that was accomplished could I start to move toward healing.

Coming to believe that Heavenly Father could restore me to complete spiritual health took some time. I was angry and distrustful. I did what everyone else has done—I asked the "why" question. Why didn't He stop the abuse? For a while, no answers came. Yes, He was there in the counseling sessions, and He definitely led the therapy. His hand guided and directed the counselor and myself. Tiny miracles happened repeatedly in those offices. Yet I did not receive answers to my "why" questions.

Over time, my questions changed. In my prayers, I started asking that my experience would not be for nothing. I wanted something good to come from all the pain and heartache. I asked Heavenly Father if, because of my pain, I might be able to help others in their pain. Repeatedly, this prayer has been answered and the request fulfilled.

Elder Orson F. Whitney of the Council of the Twelve reflected on one possible reason terrible things happen to us. He said, "To whom do we look, in days of grief and disaster, for help and consolation? . . . They are men and women who have suffered, and out of their experience in suffering they bring forth the riches of their sympathy and condolences as a blessing to those now in need. Could they do this had they not suffered themselves? . . . Is not this God's purpose in causing his children to suffer? He wants them to become more like himself. God has suffered far more than man ever did or ever will, and is therefore the great source of sympathy and consolation" (Whitney, 1918).

This, in large part, answered my why question. I slowly began to feel God's love for me. I could feel His Spirit, the Holy Ghost, comforting me as though God Himself was holding me. This is what built my hope and faith. This is what lifted my spirits. I dared to dream I could be made whole. I was like a fractured piece of glass, broken into a bunch of jagged shards. How could anyone put me back together as a whole person?

I have to admit, there is no easy way. There has been no shortcut, nothing less than walking the hard path that brought me to healing. I am grateful for the journey. I confess that I sometimes acted like Laman and Lemuel. And there has often been a "Nephi" counseling me, humbling me, helping me to stop fighting against the journey, and helping me believe there really was a promised land. Sometimes that Nephi figure was a bishop. Sometimes it was my wife, or my counselor, or the scriptures. And sometimes it was the Lord Himself.

I have a new-found respect for those wayward older brothers of Nephi. I had always painted Laman and Lemuel as the bad guys in the Book of Mormon. Now I see myself in their attitudes and their lack of faith. I see myself in their wanting to go back to an easier way of life, and in their complaints about how hard the journey is. I see myself in Laman and Lemuel as they struggle to understand the words of God. I see myself in how easily they forget the past miracles as soon as a new hardship comes along. I see myself in them when they see a huge roadblock and cannot fathom how things will work out. They can't seem to see beyond the problem; they get stuck in it and give up because they can see no way out. How many times have I been in that mind space?

As we move forward toward applying the Atonement in our lives, these coping skills need to be replaced. We need to practice new skills that foster living instead of surviving. Even though it may be frightening and even anxiety provoking, letting go of these deeply held coping mechanisms is essential if we want to feel the Savior's healing power in our lives. Elder Richard G. Scott of the Quorum of the Twelve Apostles reminds us that there is no shortcut in obtaining the healing miracle of the Atonement: "The beginning of healing requires childlike faith in the unalterable fact that Father in Heaven loves you and has supplied a way to heal. His Beloved Son, Jesus Christ, laid down His life to provide that healing. But there is no magic solution, no simple balm to provide healing, nor is there an easy path to the complete remedy. The cure requires profound faith in Jesus Christ and in His infinite capacity to heal. It is rooted in an understanding of doctrine and a resolute determination to follow it" (Scott, 2008).

The initial pain is over and the initial shock is gone. For most of us, the abuse happened long ago. We have had many years to practice our coping methods. Often it is the problems caused by the coping mechanisms that lead us to seek relief, not the actual abuse itself. And so, like I did with my knee, we get scheduled for "surgery." The surgery is the act of opening ourselves up to see the reality of what happened, to see the ripple effect the trauma has had in our lives, and to see how our current methods of "managing" the past are ineffective and ultimately destructive.

Let's be willing to let go, to reach out, and to trust our Savior as He teaches us new ways to cope with the wounds in our souls. Let's put the crutches down, take a deep breath, and step forward, trusting that He will be there to catch us if we start to fall. Let's trust that He knows how to heal us better than we do. The Lord does know better, and He is anxious to help.

The following assessment, developed by John Bradshaw, will help clarify how much we are using maladaptive ways to handle past traumas. This list includes attitudes, beliefs, and behaviors that people may experience when some form of childhood wounding occurred in their past. The more you see yourself in this list, the more your life is filled with stumbling blocks to accessing the Atonement—and the more you need to heal from the past. Read the following statements and answer true or false, depending on whether or not they apply to you.

- I experience anxiety and fear whenever I contemplate doing anything new.
- I am a people pleaser.
- I am a rebel. I feel alive when I'm in conflict.
- In the deepest place of my secret self, I feel there is something wrong with me.
- I'm a hoarder; I have trouble letting go of anything.
- I feel inadequate as a man/woman.
- I am confused about my sexual identity.
- I feel guilty when I stand up for myself and would rather give in to others.
- I have trouble starting things.
- I have trouble finishing things.
- I rarely think for myself.
- I continually criticize myself for being inadequate.
- I consider myself a terrible sinner and believe I will go to hell.
- I'm rigid and perfectionistic.
- I feel like I never measure up; I never get anything right.
- I feel like I really don't know what I want.
- I'm driven to be a super-achiever.
- I feel I don't really matter except when I'm sexual. I'm afraid I'll be rejected and abandoned if I'm not a good lover.

- My life is empty; I feel depressed a lot of the time.
- I don't really know who I am; I'm not sure what my values are or what I think about things.
- I'm out of touch with my physical body.
- I don't like being touched.
- I often have sex when I really don't want to.
- I currently have or have had an eating disorder.
- I am hung up on oral sex.
- I rarely know what I feel.
- I feel ashamed when I get mad.
- I feel ashamed when I get scared.
- I am ashamed when I cry.
- I fear other people's anger and will do almost anything to try to control it.
- I rarely get mad, but when I do, I rage.
- I'm obsessed with anal sex.
- I'm obsessed with sado/masochistic sex.
- I'm ashamed of my bodily functions.
- I have sleep disorders.
- I spend an inordinate amount of time looking at pornography.
- I have exhibited myself sexually in a way that violates others.
- I am sexually attracted to children and am afraid I might act it out.
- I believe that food and/or sex are my greatest needs.
- I basically distrust everyone, including myself.
- I have been or am now married to an addict.
- I am obsessive and controlling in my relationship.
- I am an addict.
- I'm isolating and afraid of people, especially authority figures.

- I hate being alone and will do almost anything to avoid it.
- I find myself doing what I think others expect me to do.
- I avoid conflict at all cost.
- I have an overdeveloped sense of responsibility. It is easier for me to be concerned with others than with myself.
- I often do not say no directly but then I refuse, in indirect and manipulative ways, to do what others have asked.
- I don't know how to resolve conflicts. I am either overpowering or completely passive.
- I never felt close to one or both of my parents.
- I confuse love with pity and tend to love people I can pity.
- I ridicule myself and others if a mistake is made.
- I give in easily.
- I'm a fierce competitor and a poor loser.
- My most profound fear is that of abandonment and I'll do anything to hold onto a relationship. (Bradshaw, 1990)

If ten or more of the preceding statements are true for you, you need to access the Atonement and heal from your past.

CHAPTER 6
HOLDING FAST

It was 1988, and I was stationed in the city of Luxemburg, in the tiny country of Luxemburg. It was my first area while serving in the Belgium Brussels Mission. Only three families came to church. There were no other Latter-day Saints—no less-active members to visit, no "lost" members, not even any part-member families to work with. Every day we focused on finding new investigators. Every day we tracted and did street contacting, for twelve hours a day. I still struggled to speak and understand French. In my four months in Luxemburg, we taught a total of seven lessons, two of which I slept through. To say that this type of mission life crushed my hope and optimism would be an understatement.

During my time in Luxemburg, I had a very realistic dream. To this day, I can recall it with clarity. I can see the colors, feel the way I felt when I first had the dream, and remember the tiniest details. Perhaps it was more than just a dream. In the dream I was in a large city, lining up with many other people for a marathon. The gun fired, and everybody started running. I quickly dropped to the back of the group. The day was sunny and the path was clearly marked. As I ran, I saw fewer and fewer people. The day turned to night and I still ran, trying to finish.

As the night wore on, it became harder and harder to follow the outlined path. Then a heavy fog rolled in. Now it was dark and foggy. I could barely see in front of me. I slowed down and watched carefully to make sure I didn't take a wrong turn and leave the marathon route. By this point, I was so tired I don't know if what I was doing could actually be called running. It looked more like staggering. My mouth was dry, my lips were cracked, and I needed water badly. The muscles in my legs were screaming for me to stop. I stayed committed, however, and kept going. I remained in this state for what seemed like forever. By now I wasn't even thinking about finishing the race. I wasn't even thinking about why I wanted to do this marathon or who was rooting for me. I couldn't see anybody because of the fog. Ever step I took felt as though I was running on broken ankles.

Finally, I could take no more. I collapsed on the road, raised my hand, and whispered, "I give up. I'm done." Suddenly the fog lifted. I could see the street lights again, and their brilliance showed the path clearly. And there, no more than three feet away, was the finish line. I was three feet from finishing this most grueling race. I had given everything I had, but had quit three feet from the finish line. Suddenly the exhaustion and physical pain disappeared. Instead I was filled with a sense of regret and disappointment so profound that these feelings stayed with me days after the dream. How could I have given up just three feet from the finish line? It didn't seem to matter anymore that I couldn't see the finish line when I gave up. It didn't matter that I had no more strength when I gave up. All that I could see was that the finish line was a lousy three feet from where I collapsed and quit.

The dream came back to me several more times, and each time left me feeling haunted with a sense of profound regret. Decades past and that dream periodically popped into my mind. In the midst of fighting to overcome my own past, I related the dream to my bishop. His eyes lit up and he seemed very interested. He eagerly listened to my account and then started searching for a scripture.

"Your dream reminds me of Lehi's dream. People in his dream tried to follow a path. They encountered a heavy fog, and it was difficult for them to keep going." My bishop pointed out key words Lehi used to describe what it was like for these people—"pressing forward," "caught hold," "clinging to the rod of iron," "continually holding fast to the rod of iron" (1 Nephi 8:21–30).

As the bishop related Lehi's dream to mine, I suddenly understood my dream in a new way. This was a dream about my journey to find healing. The dream's message underscored the idea that if I relied on myself, I would indeed expend a great deal of energy and see progress made, but would be unable to find that lasting peace I was looking for.

In fact, I had spent thousands of hours in recovery support groups. I had tried acupuncture, EMDR, guided imagery, and yoga. I had read scores of books, checked myself into an inpatient facility, and over the course of my journey worked with over ten different therapists. I tried meditation, reiki healing, and music therapy with imbedded brain waves. I participated in psychodrama and affirmation exercises. I took Epsom salt baths. I do not discount anything I tried, as each of the methods and techniques offered me something and blessed me with insight that helped me understand myself better. What remained elusive was the sense of being free from the past. And now, in the bishop's office, he was showing me the missing piece of the dream—how to finish the race.

"See the words Lehi uses?" he asked me. "These are action words. These words show the desperate place these people were in and how they clung to the rod of iron as if it was their lifeline. They were not passive—casually leaning on a banister, or letting go periodically to wander around. They clung. They held fast. So when hard times come and you want to return to your old coping methods, hold fast. Hold fast to the iron rod and you will finish the race, victorious."

I left the bishop's office with that short phrase buzzing in my head: "Hold fast." Holding fast to the iron rod will help me better connect to the Atonement. It will open my heart to let the Holy Ghost comfort me, inspire me, soothe me, and sanctify me. Holding fast will help me remain steadfast even when it seems as the gates of hell are gaping open to destroy me. As Elder Kevin S. Hamilton of the Seventy explained, "The rod of iron represented . . . the only safety and security that they could find, and they held fast continually; they refused to let go" (Hamilton, 2014).

Holding fast to the scriptures, to Heavenly Father, to the Savior's words of encouragement—these are the anchors when the storms come. These are the lifelines to making it through the dark and stormy night. And even when we don't see or feel the Lord reaching out to us (just like the mist in Lehi's dream hid the tree of life from view—making it hard to experience the love of God) we hold fast. Even when I can't run another step in my dream, I hold fast. And help will come. Sometimes quickly and miraculously, sometimes slowly, but I have found it always comes.

Overcoming past childhood abuse, no matter the form, is filled with many starts and stops and even some full-on face plants. After all, we're trying to heal our relationships with our Heavenly Father and our Savior, trying to understand our coping skills that have become dysfunctional, and trying to learn new ways to handle the stress and anxiety that used to trigger us—all at the same time. Yet there is hope.

The Atonement allows us to get back up when we're stumbling and try again. In April 2015 general conference, Elder Dale G. Renlund of the First Quorum of the Seventy said:

> *In less formal terms, God cares a lot more about who we are and who we are becoming than about who we once were. He cares that we keep on trying. . . . President Thomas S. Monson has taught,*

> *"One of God's greatest gifts to us is the joy of trying again, for no failure ever need be final" (Thomas S. Monson, "The Will Within," Ensign, May 1987). . . . The Savior's infinite Atonement can heal even, and perhaps especially, those who have innocently suffered. He understands perfectly what it is like to suffer innocently as a consequence of another's transgression. As prophesied, the Savior will "bind up the brokenhearted . . . give . . . beauty for ashes, the oil of joy for mourning, [and] the garment of praise for the spirit of heaviness" (Isaiah 61:1–3). No matter what, with His help, God expects Latter-day Saints to keep on trying.* (Renlund, 2015)

The rest of this book will teach you how to access the healing, freeing power of the Savior's Atonement as you try to overcome your traumatic past. As you work through these past abuses, hold fast. Your faith may be tried. Hold fast. Your nights might be troubled with nightmares and flashbacks. Hold fast. You may feel overwhelmed and drained. Hold fast.

Please try. Just try. And as Elder Renlund counseled, keep trying. Sometimes trying simply looks like showing up. Sometimes trying is just continuing to take your anti-depressants as prescribed. Sometimes trying is reading one verse of scripture. Sometimes trying is picking up a phone to reach out to a friend. Sometimes it looks like snuggling with your husband or wife. Sometimes it looks like taking a soak in the tub, or sipping hot soup. Keep trying, no matter how tiny the effort is. Hold fast, even if all you can do is imagine you are holding fast.

We will win the race. We will taste of the fruit of the tree of life. We will break free of the chains that bind us. We will one day feel the lasting peace that solid healing brings. Along the way, hold fast.

Part 2

Attachment and the Atonement

But now thus saith the Lord that created thee, O Jacob, and he that formed thee, O Israel, Fear not: for I have redeemed thee, I have called thee by thy name; thou art mine. When thou passest through the waters, I will be with thee; and through the rivers, they shall not overflow thee: when thou walkest through the fire, thou shalt not be burned; neither shall the flame kindle upon thee. —Isaiah 43:1–2

Chapter 7
Session with Terri

It was a rainy, wintry day—pretty normal for the Pacific Northwest. I sat down and motioned for Terri to sit as well. She didn't look good. Her black hair seemed dull and flat. The dark circles under her eyes accentuated the unusual paleness of her face. It looked as though she was wearing her pajamas and hadn't showered yet. She had called me around eleven the night before, crying hysterically. She was terrified to go to sleep, not wanting to have another flashback.

"You don't look good," I said to her.

She grunted. "I don't feel very good."

"As a matter of fact, you look terrible."

Smiling, she gave a short laugh. "Aren't you supposed to be helping me with my self-esteem?" I laughed with her. She needed a little humor.

"How did the night go after we hung up?" I asked.

Terri curled up on the couch, tucking her feet in tight against herself. "I didn't really sleep," she said, then pulled her hair back and put it in a ponytail.

"So let's review a bit," I began. "A flashback is our body's way of telling its story. It's like a piece of glacier that breaks off from the bottom and floats to the surface. We don't always know what is happening, and the incoming sensory input doesn't match what is actually going on in the moment."

"Like when I was eating dinner the other night."

I nodded. Two nights previously, Terri had experienced a flashback at the dinner table. Suddenly she couldn't move or speak. Her husband said her eyes got huge and her mouth opened up wide, but she didn't scream. He quickly took the kids into another room. Several minutes past where Terri remained in that fixed position. When she could move again, she slumped onto the dining room table, breathing heavily. Soon afterward, she experienced a severe headache and went to bed.

"Flashbacks can happen in any of several different ways," I said. "We can feel an intense emotion that we felt during the abuse. Or images come to us, like still pictures, or bits and pieces of memories. Some people actually experience the physical sensations of the abuse. Others experience auditory, visual, physical, and emotional feelings, as if the abuse was happening that instant."

"Like they were reliving it?" Terri asked.

"Yes."

"I didn't see anything in my head. I didn't feel like the abuse was happening. I was just suddenly frozen with intense fear," she explained.

"Like when you realized you were trapped in the evil clown's storage compartment."

Terri nodded, a faraway look in her eyes as if she was recalling that terrible event. "Until that point, I didn't know he was a bad man. I thought we were going to his garage to look at his clown stuff. I had no idea what was going to happen."

"Of course not. You were five. And this guy had only been nice to you up until this moment. You had no reason to suspect anything. How could you have known his secret intentions?"

"When I first met him, he smiled at me and gave me some cookies. Mom didn't like me eating cookies. I told him that. He said we could eat them together and keep it a special secret." Terri was whispering and almost seemed to be in a trance state. Suddenly a shiver went through her body and she looked at me, refocusing. "I thought he was a nice man," she said with an edge to her voice.

"He wanted you to think that."

She frowned and her eyes narrowed. "I was innocent and he took advantage of that!" she said angrily.

"Yes."

"He took away my ability to trust others!"

"Yes," I said.

"I'll never let that happen to me again!"

"Right, because you should have known."

"Yeah!" Terri agreed.

"You should have seen this coming."

"Yeah!"

"You should have never gotten into his car."

"Right!"

Taking a risk, I said, "It was all your fault."

"Yes!" she exclaimed.

And then there was silence. It took Terri a moment to realize what she had just said. I waited, looking expectantly at her. She glanced at me questioningly. Seeing the gears turning in her head, I nodded and smiled slightly.

"I've blamed myself for the abuse all this time," she whispered so softly I barely heard her. Her expression changed with a sense of awareness.

Remaining silent, I motioned for her to keep going.

"So not only am I never going to trust ever again, I'm bad and stupid for even allowing the clown man to rape me." More connections were being made as Terri spoke out loud. This was new territory for her.

"And because of this belief, you can't even begin to imagine that God would want you," I said.

She nodded. "Yeah. That's why I worked so hard as a missionary. I had to prove to God that I wasn't a piece of garbage. I had to prove to Him that I wasn't bad or stupid."

"And it is why, when you pray, you second-guess yourself. How can you give yourself to God when you can't trust people's intentions? Maybe God is lying. Maybe He really wants to get you and damn you. Maybe He has ulterior motives."

Terri gave a short laugh. "What are you saying, that I see God the same way as I see the clown man? That's terrible!"

I didn't respond, just raised my eyebrows.

"God isn't going to hurt me," Terri scoffed. "He loves me."

"How do you feel when He loves you?" I asked.

She screwed up her face. "Why do you say it like that?"

"Like what?"

"Like that—like He's loving me romantically."

"I didn't say God was loving you romantically. I was simply asking what your experience was like when you felt His love." I paused. "But maybe you just answered that question."

Terri scratched her head nervously. Her feet were no longer curled up, but were tapping on the floor.

"When someone says they love you, what do you think they mean by that?"

"That they love me." She shrugged nervously.

"And what do people do when they love someone?" I asked carefully.

Terri chewed on the inside of her cheek. Her knee was bouncing so fast, I could feel it in my chair. She muttered something about her uncle that I couldn't understand. Suddenly she exploded up off the couch. She pointed a finger at me and yelled, "They take you and they rape you! All they want is to have sex with you!"

I nodded, remaining very still. Terri started to pace around in the office.

After watching her for a few moments, I asked, "Why are you pacing?"

"Because I can't sit still right now," she snapped.

"Well, can you pace faster?"

"Of course I can."

"Can you pace slower?"

"Nope."

"Can you pace just around the couch?"

"Yeah," she looked at me, clearly puzzled and irritated.

"Well, what about pacing in a small circle?"

Terri stopped pacing. "What are you doing?"

"I'm trying to get you to pace with purpose."

"Why?"

"Because then you will be more grounded, more 'here,' more in control."

Terri sat down, shaking her head. "You are a nut case," she muttered.

"And you have just proven why trying to do what the bishop is asking you to do doesn't work. You can't trust God when He says He loves you. You can't be 100% certain that He will always be honest and forthright with you. You can't allow yourself to be vulnerable with Him because that would open you up to be abused again."

Terri stared at me for a few moments, gave a big sigh, and sank deeper into the couch. "How could I not see that?" she finally asked.

"You formed a lot of these beliefs when you were abused. And just like it's not easy for you to think about the abuse, it is equally difficult to uncover the foundational beliefs caused by the abuse." I lean forward. "Terri, look at me. Heavenly Father is nothing like any man you have ever met on earth. He is not like any of your abusers. He isn't even anything like your own dad. Every example you have of what a man is, doesn't fit with how Heavenly Father acts. He is safe. His love is pure. He is 100% straightforward and honest. Remember, the scriptures state that He can't lie. He can't deceive. The Apostle John said that God is love, because He loves us so much."

The Spirit filled the room as I began to testify of Heavenly Father's love for all of His children. Terri stared at me spellbound. She gulped and put her hand to her chest. I nodded slowly and told her it was okay.

"This is His love, Terri. This is Him letting you know He loves you." I paused, watching her closely. She swallowed again, breathed heavily, and closed her eyes. She whispered to herself, "This is safe. This is safe. This is safe."

"Yes, Terri. God is safe."

Chapter 8
Attachment and the Atonement

When we were children, how our parents reacted toward us shaped our beliefs about ourselves—whether or not we were valuable and worthwhile. What a child believes becomes his or her reality, since the child has no ability to "bounce" ideas off others. If a parent is easily irritated and frustrated by the child's knocking over the milk for the second time that day, the child quickly incorporates the idea that as a person he or she is a nuisance and an irritant. Children who come to see themselves as problems tend to have trouble believing in a God that is loving and not out to punish them.

Maltreated children expect situations to confirm what they have learned in their relationships with their maltreating parent(s). When experiences with God are contrary to these expectations, even if the experiences are positive, anxiety escalates (Anderson, 2005). Clearly, the style of attachment we experienced as children directly impacts the way we come to see ourselves and the type of relationship we have with God. All the more reason to hold fast to the gospel while we ride the wave of anxiety and uncertainty. Eventually, repeated positive experiences with Heavenly Father will create a new set of expectations, and anxiety will decrease.

What is attachment? Attachment bonds have at least three key elements: "One, an attachment bond is an enduring emotional relationship with a specific person; two, the relationship brings safety, comfort, soothing, and pleasure; and three, the loss or threat of loss of the person evokes intense distress" (Perry, 1999). Attachment, however, does not happen just during infancy or early childhood. There will always be times in life where we seek out others to receive soothing support and allow ourselves to be vulnerable. Often whom we turn to is a reflection of the type of attachment we had as infants with our parents.

Life is hard. We live in a mortal, fallen world. As one colleague often says, "This world is a dangerous neighborhood." Most parents are not overtly, consciously trying to damage their son or daughter. They are doing the best they can with what they have. And sometimes, there isn't that much to give.

For example, a mother has three children under the age of five and the newborn is colicky. Attachment is going to be difficult. The mother doesn't mean to or want to have trouble attaching to her new baby. Maybe the mother suffers from post-partum depression. The child is going to have trouble attaching to a depressed person. The mother can't control it—depression after pregnancy is a part of life for some women. For others, their mother will have struggled with depression even before getting pregnant.

Perhaps the child was born to a father who can't control his anger. He struggles to control his rage and is very impatient. He doesn't want to hurt his child, but after the child cries for ten minutes, dumping the child in a room and slamming the door is the only thing the father can do. If that happens enough, the child will learn that having needs is dangerous—it equals being rejected and abandoned.

Many children are born to parents who are much more damaged—alcoholics, meth users, prescription drug abusers. Some parents are physically, emotionally, and sexually abusive. There is clear evidence that traumatic and abusive experiences inhibit a person's ability to attach securely and positively with others.

Psychologically, there are a host of beliefs and messages that restrict an individual from having a successful life full of rich and rewarding relationships. Biologically, the body changes and adapts to trauma and abuse such that balance and regulation are severely hampered. What remains is a series of maladaptive coping skills aimed at overcoming the emotional, mental, and physical deficits of poor attachment. These dysfunctional attachment skills easily become addictive both psychologically and physically. As such, the ability to develop and grow is limited.

In the end, everyone is raised by imperfect people in a fallen world. No one escapes childhood without some bumps and bruises, emotionally as well as physically. Some people leave childhood with deeper scars than others. Some grow into adulthood with their childhood wounds still feeling fresh, raw, and open. Everyone, though, carries something from the past. Everyone.

I worked with a man named Rex who had attachment issues, having been raised in an emotionally and sexually incestuous home. One exercise I had him do was to allow that hurting, scared part of him that didn't trust anyone to write a story. It is rich in metaphor. The story shows the changes in thinking he went through to survive living in such a dysfunctional home. Notice how this part of Rex's psyche sees his parent as a crafty monster, and the evolving relationship he had with this monster.

> *One day Johnny wanted to go swimming in the river behind his house. He was really excited. He ran off the deck and jumped into the water. As Johnny was swimming, he got swallowed up by a big green monster. He was safe because he was in a bubble in the monster's stomach. The monster burped and the bubble shot out of the monster's mouth. Johnny was free!*
>
> *But the monster was sad. It didn't have any friends. Johnny said, "I'll be your friend, but you can't eat me, okay?" The*

monster was happy and promised not to eat Johnny. After they played for a while, the monster got hungry. "Could I eat just your hand? That's all . . . I promise."

Johnny said, "Okay," as long as it was just his hand. The hand tasted really good. Pretty soon the monster begged and begged to eat the other hand. Johnny got tired of the monster asking, so he finally said, "Okay." It didn't hurt that bad.

Now that Johnny didn't have any hands, he had to have the monster pick things up for him. After a while the monster ate Johnny's left leg when Johnny wasn't looking. Johnny was having fun in the water, riding the monster's tail.

Before long, the monster had eaten Johnny's legs, shoulders, and stomach. By this time, Johnny forgot what it felt like to have a body. He was happy to still have his head. Then the monster threw Johnny in the air and gulped down his head.

This story is about the sneaky monster. Remember, monsters can never be trusted. No matter how nice they are, all they really want to do is eat you.

Below is a list of parental behaviors and attitudes that can negatively impact a child's attachment and self-esteem. A child doesn't have to be physically or sexually abused to experience trauma. This list is not all-inclusive, but it is meant to get you thinking about how your parents treated, interacted with, and parented you.

- Cold and distant, aloof
- Superficially charming
- Rigid, high expectations
- Lack of mercy and forgiveness
- Constantly busy—a doer
- Depressed

- Extremely religious and judgmental
- Chronically ill
- Alcoholic or drug addict
- Two faced—acted one way in public, another way in private
- Preachy and fault finding
- Sex addict
- Easily overwhelmed, easily frustrated, rage outbursts
- Physically abusive, emotionally abusive, or sexually abusive
- Extremely affectionate to the point of making others uncomfortable
- Rarely held you accountable
- Easily manipulated, naive
- Little or no rules, little structure
- Impulsive, controlling, mood swings—very manic to very depressed
- Overly involved, love/hate relationship with you
- Denied you privacy
- Wanted to keep you dependent—not allowing you to grow up

Understanding the way you attach and bond with others (and yourself) is key in making necessary changes and in letting go of old, stuck patterns that no longer work. This is what builds and supports a person's sense of inner/personal power. It creates freedom and peace, and it allows the individual to accept love and give love. This awareness will truly help bring about healing.

The next four chapters will review the four basic types of attachment and how they impact our spiritual relationship with Heavenly Father and Jesus Christ. See if you can find yourself in any of these attachment styles.

CHAPTER 9
SECURE ATTACHMENT

Research in the field of attachment disorder focuses on four major forms of attaching to another person. The first category, and the healthiest style, is that of secure attachment. These are secure adults who were raised in a consistent, reliable, and caring way. An estimated 55% to 65% of children experience a secure attachment to their primary caregiver. They exhibit a basic understanding of how to integrate experiences into their lives.

The Secure Attachment Style

Secure attachment exhibits the following characteristics:

The primary caregiver

- Is attuned to the infant / toddler / child / adolescent
- Reflects back what the infant / toddler / child / adolescent is feeling; often holds the child's gaze, makes cooing and loving noises to the infant / toddler; is physically affectionate
- Is consistent and reliable in terms of behaviors, reactions, and adherence to rules

The child (now an adult)

- Has a realistic sense of danger and often uses social supports to help manage crises

- Shows a balance between relying on self and asking others for help
- Exhibits a wide range of coping skills—both cognitive and emotional, mental and behavioral
- Is less at risk for developing serious mental health issues such as chronic PTSD (Goldberg, 2004)

Attachment styles are the template for current and future relationships, including our relationships with our Heavenly Father and Savior Jesus Christ. These styles will impact how we relate to, connect with, and think about our Heavenly Parents, our Elder Brother Jesus Christ, and the Holy Ghost. The more secure we feel in our relationships with our mortal, earthly parents, the more we will feel secure with Heavenly Father. Let's review, then, the impact a secure attachment will have on our spirituality.

The Spiritually Secure Attachment Style

Individuals who have a spiritually secure attachment are prone to do the following:

- See God as trustworthy, loving, caring, and compassionate
- Find it easier to be humble and penitent; feel safe being vulnerable with God
- Rarely second guess when praying to God; have a sense of how Heavenly Father communicates with them; trust the promptings of the Holy Spirit
- Feel comfortable and comforted with seeing God as a Father; do not fear reaching out to Him
- Celebrate the Atonement, rather than shunning it or feeling guilty about using it
- Rely on God, believing nothing can damage the love the Father and the Son have for them

Secure attachment does not mean the individual experiences no trials or hardships. It doesn't even necessarily preclude experiencing abuse outside of the home. What sets the securely attached adult apart from other attachment styles is the relationship between the adult as a child and his or her parents. Parents who help form a secure attachment with their children have developed a specific set of skills.

Patience and long-suffering is one of the most important traits to foster within oneself in order to be a healthy parent, for obvious reasons. There are countless occasions when a child will test and try the patience of his or her parents. Why? Because children do not possess the ability to self-regulate. They require outside help to contain, manage, and learn how to process emotions. They require assistance to manage cravings and urges. They need help to learn how to self-soothe, and over time, how to be okay with delayed gratification.

If you, as a parent, do not know how to do those things for yourself, it is nearly impossible to teach your children how to do them. Remember the adage "You can't give what you don't have." As much as children will listen to their parents, what they actually emulate is the parents' behavior, attitudes, reactions to stress, and overall spiritual conditions. Children are biologically created to be attuned to all the unspoken messages of their parents. Therefore, as a parent, what type of an individual you are is more important than what you say.

In *Healing the Codependent Heart* (2013), I wrote about and explored charity-based parenting. The more parents can implement the concept of charity into their daily interactions with their children, the more likely they are to foster a secure attachment with their offspring. In Moroni 7:45 we read, "And charity suffereth long, and is kind, and envieth not, and is not puffed up, seeketh not her own, is not easily provoked, thinketh no evil, and rejoiceth not in iniquity but rejoiceth in the truth, beareth all things, believeth all things, hopeth all things, endureth all things."

If you do not possess all these qualities, begin now to incorporate them. Practice them. Learn how to apply them in your daily parenting struggles. It is never too late to learn how to be a healthy, Christ-centered parent.

CHAPTER 10

AVOIDANT/ANXIOUS ATTACHMENT

The second category of attachment bonding is avoidant adults, who were raised by unnurturing, dismissive, and critical parents. Approximately 20% to 25% of children experience an avoidant attachment to their primary caregiver. Parents of avoidant adults were usually emotionally controlling. In turn, the child grew up believing that emotional-based information is highly unreliable and even dangerous. Avoidant adults are often uncomfortable with closeness and intimacy. They have trouble asking for help. They are often passive-aggressive and lean toward a heavy dependency on intellect. Often, they use the pronoun "you" instead of "I" when talking about themselves. Furthermore, these adults find it difficult to integrate information from the past with the present (Cochrane, 2003).

The Avoidant Attachment Style

Individuals who have an avoidant attachment have a tendency to do the following:

- Deny danger and minimize trauma
- Distrust others' help
- Cope via distraction and withdrawal
- Numb their "negative" feelings
- Use avoidant and passive coping strategies

- Overestimate their own strength in terms of being able to handle traumatic stressors
- Dismiss emotional needs to avoid closeness
- See their parents as not responding to their needs; learn to rely on themselves
- Distrust their own emotions
- Can be seen as hostile and anti-social; may hurt others
- Focus attention on non-human things—TV, video games, fixing the house, cleaning the car, etc. (Goldberg, 2004)

The avoidant template is most often formed when emotional/verbal abuse is experienced. Shirley Glass (2003) explains that individuals who experienced avoidant bonding with their primary caregivers often see marriage as confining. Affairs are seen as a way to get space. These individuals fear being vulnerable, and they struggle to open up.

Those who are avoidant act overly independent. The template may look something like this: Emotional closeness isn't safe. If I open up and become vulnerable, I will get hurt.

The Spiritually Avoidant Attachment Style

Spiritually, the avoidant individual can come across as willful and stubborn. However, these attributes can have positive aspects. A willful person doesn't usually give up. A willful person doesn't care about stumbling blocks; he or she will find a way to get around the blockage. Being stubborn can also mean a person is committed to his or her point of view. If that point of view is the same as God's, then the person is usually rock solid. A stubborn person is a fighter and a survivor, and he or she can be doggedly persistent. The goal is to help the avoidant individual feel safe and then work with that person to shift his or her focus to be aligned with God's purposes.

People with a spiritually avoidant attachment are likely to:

- Struggle to pray—prefer to handle a situation or problem alone; don't want to "bother" God with their issues
- See God as dismissive, cold, and distant; believe they have to "earn" His love
- Believe they must be perfect in order to gain God's love and access the Atonement
- Believe God is looking to punish them
- Struggle to be open and vulnerable with God
- Keep the Atonement far away, seeing it as unfair; want to suffer for their own sins rather than having Christ suffer for them

At the core, the spiritually avoidant person has low self-esteem. Love has been experienced as conditional. Therefore, the person feels he or she is not good enough to be loved or validated. This idea must be attacked head on. Over and over and over, the case must be made to the avoidant person that Heavenly Father loves him or her, regardless of the individual's past behavior. The person needs to come to believe that his or her worth and value exist independently of his or her actions. Nothing the person does can make him or her less or more in the eyes of God. Sometimes it seems as though a sledgehammer is needed to pound away at these twisted and distorted beliefs that are woven into the avoidant person's foundation.

It takes humility to access Christ's suffering on our behalf. The avoidant individual will need to unravel any kind of shame that prevents him or her from accepting the Atonement. Since love is seen as conditional, most avoidant adults believe they are worthless because they are not perfect. Shame is often at the core of their personalities. And this type of shame doesn't produce remorse or a desire to change. In fact, this type of shame creates negative pride—where people see themselves as so bad that not even Christ can save them.

Case Story

Ann sat next to Juan. He and I had been working together for over a year. They were engaged to be married, but he was having trouble believing she would stay with him. He had a string of failed relationships before he met her, and in every case his girlfriend had cheated on him. He believed Ann would do the same.

Juan had been abandoned by his mother and raised by relatives until age three, whereupon Mom suddenly showed up and took him back. She regularly picked her other children over Juan, taking their side and meeting their needs and desires before his, often leaving him alone at home while she and the rest of the family went on vacations.

I instructed Ann to snuggle up to Juan, put her hand on his chest, and whisper that she loved him. While she did this, I asked Juan to lay back, breathe deeply, and imagine that he was opening up the doors to his heart for Ann. He struggled at first, turning his head back and forth. His fists were clenched.

"You can do this, Juan," I said gently. "Ann has proven she is safe. She isn't going anywhere." She continued to whisper that she loved him and gently caressed his chest. "Imagine those walls you have built to keep your heart safe, slowly coming down," I said.

He started to hyperventilate. "Breathe, Juan, from your belly like we practiced," I said, trying to coach him through the moment.

In a broken sob, he cried out, "No!"

"Juan, Ann loves you," I encouraged. "You love Ann. Let her love in."

Suddenly he exploded in wave after wave of sobs. His body was racked with these full-body cries of pain and hurt. Ann continued to hold him and whisper that she loved him. This incredible unleashing continued for several minutes. Slowly his sobbing became weeping, and his weeping turned to periodic gushes of breath escaping from his mouth.

He opened his eyes. Ann looked up at him expectantly. He wiped his eyes and then broke into a smile. "I can feel her love! It's awesome!" He hugged her and she hugged him. They stayed like that for several minutes. I sat back with tears in my own eyes, remembering a similar experience I had with my own wife. How glorious it is to finally connect to another's love!

A month later, I attended their wedding. It was small and simple, but the two of them were beaming. Their future looked bright. Learning to open up to Ann's love allowed Juan to feel Christ's love. Now he could begin to heal from the damaging, soul-tearing experience of being routinely abandoned by his family.

The Anxious Attachment Style

Associated with the avoidant form of attachment is its shadow or opposite—the anxious adult. This template sounds something like "I crave love. There is nothing as bottomless as is my craving to love and be loved." Even if the person remains mostly in one state (avoidant) or the other (anxious), an undercurrent of the other extreme will always be present.

Individuals with an anxious attachment are prone to:

- Be overly insecure about their relationships
- Have a greater need for emotional closeness than their partners
- Fear abandonment
- Base their self-worth on feedback from others
- Struggle with anxiety
- Be people pleasers, overly focused on others' needs

- (If affairs and emotional acting out occur) Act obsessively and intensely; connections happen almost instantaneously

People with anxious attachments can be prone to hide their sins, as they don't want others to see their weaknesses and reject them. The anxious individual will appear very willing to help. However, his or her motivation (even if it is hidden or subconscious) comes from a deep well of fear. Nothing motivates an anxious adult more than the fear of being abandoned. Love and acceptance always hinges on the last great moment of success.

The Spiritually Anxious Attachment Style

Individuals with a spiritually anxious attachment tend to:

- Constantly wonder if they are good enough to merit God's love and blessings; see His love as conditional
- Fear incurring God's wrath; feel more worried about being rejected by God than by being loved by Him
- Be "doers" in the congregation, but the motivation is often based on fear rather than on love
- Struggle to believe God will really forgive them, even if the Spirit confirms it or the bishop declares it
- Question the answers they receive from God, and struggle when prayers are not immediately answered
- Show a lack of faith and trust in God due to fear
- Be perfectionists, believing one mistake means God no longer loves them.

What someone with an anxious attachment needs to work on is faith—faith in God, faith in the concept of real love, and faith in himself or herself. Fear needs to be addressed and recognized in every aspect of the anxious person's relationships with others.

Having lived in a state of fear for so long, the anxious adult may not always be able to see its impact in his or her life.

And how does one overcome fear? As the Apostle John taught, "Perfect love casteth out all fear" (1 John 4:18). The only place where one can find perfect love is from the Godhead—Heavenly Father, Jesus Christ, and the Holy Ghost. Any and all distorted beliefs that relate to love need to be exhumed from the buried foundation of someone's life. In this very elementary place of one's personality lie the artifacts that have tied love and fear together.

It is not simply a fear of love that an anxious adult will exhibit; it is the fear of *losing* that love. Everything is tenuous when it comes to love. It is frail and fragile, and the slightest breeze can send it floating away, out of reach. That is why perfectionism rules the anxious individual. The fewer mistakes made, the greater the chance love will stay. This, of course, is not true.

The scriptures are replete with statements from Christ about how He loves the sinner, the imperfect, the downtrodden, and those who have been cast out. He says over and over how His hands are outstretched—waiting, begging, pleading for us to turn to Him. Perfection isn't and never has been a requirement for reaching out and receiving Christ's love.

Case Story

Carla was raised in a very chaotic home. Her parents argued constantly and often left the house in explosive fits of rage, saying they were never coming back. Throwing around the threat of divorce was common. Carla froze with fear whenever her parents started to argue. She became obsessed with the idea that if she was a really, really good girl, she could somehow ease the tension and stress at home and make Mommy and Daddy happy. Carla quickly embraced the world of the perfectionist. She studied hard, was strictly obedient, and tried to be loving to everyone she met.

By the time she married Dan, she was so entrenched in the lives of her parents and siblings that she treated her husband like a second-class citizen. Nothing was more important than staying connected to her parents. Somehow, as long as she was there, Carla believed she could keep things smooth and happy.

Eventually, her marriage started to fall apart. Dan talked about leaving. Suddenly, Carla woke up and realized she was going to lose her own marriage. She begged and sobbed for days at a time, asking Dan to stay. She owned every dysfunctional part of their marriage—even those mistakes he had made. She listened in on his phone calls and read his diary. She could barely sleep. She grilled and interrogated him when he came home from work five minutes late. She was sure he was having an affair. After all, who could love her? Why would Dan want an overweight crybaby?

In therapy, Carla would cry and often teeter on the edge of a total breakdown. She felt so overcome with fear of Dan leaving that she eventually shut down. She turned everything off and felt nothing.

As we tried to unravel this intense, paralyzing fear, I asked her how old she was. At first she gave me a quizzical look and then told me she was 47. Then I asked her if she knew how to drive a car. Yes, she replied. Did she know how to use a computer, answer a phone, or buy groceries? She answered yes to all those questions. Did she have a job? She replied that I knew she had a job, and wondered why I was asking all these silly questions.

"Before I tell you, I want you to take a deep breath, from your stomach like I taught you, and connect to that fear. Now how old do you feel?" She closed her eyes, settled into her chair a bit more, and took a deep breath. After a moment, she opened her eyes and said, "Four, maybe five years old."

"And could a four- or five-year-old live on their own?"

"No."

"What would happen to a little girl if her parents left her?"

"She would curl up and die," Carla whispered, tears welling up in her eyes.

"You think if Dan leaves you, you will die."

Carla nodded her head. "Yes. Yes, it's true."

"But you are not four or five years old. You are forty-seven. You can drive a car, buy groceries, and make money. You will continue to live even if Dan leaves you. You need to remember how old you are. This fear is not a present-based fear. This fear has been with you since early childhood. You are not a little girl anymore. You will survive if Dan leaves you."

With time, Carla overcame her fear. As she did so, she was more assertive and stopped being the scapegoat for all the problems in the marriage. She was able to tell her story and put the responsibility of her parents' marriage back with them. She started to support and choose her husband over her own family. Dan started to re-engage in the relationship. Eventually they both recommitted to the marriage.

I asked her once what it was that had helped her overcome her fear. She said simply, "Prayer."

"What do you mean? You prayed before. You went to the temple before. You got priesthood blessings. You counseled with your husband and the bishop. What is different about prayer now?"

Carla thought for a moment. "I think I was so afraid to acknowledge the fear in the first place, that I wasn't able to let God do what He needed to. I kept that part of me hidden. I wanted Him to help me, but I didn't want to open any doors that had been locked. It was like everything I had been doing was only surface deep. I had to open those doors and let Christ heal me from the inside out. Now, when I pray, I feel a connection to Heavenly Father that I have never felt before. It is healing and comforting. I believe God loves me, and I don't have to be perfect for Him to show that love to me."

Chapter 11

Ambivalent Attachment

Next is the category of ambivalent adults. Approximately 10% to 15% of all children experience an ambivalent attachment to their primary caregiver. High emotional responses seemed to be the only way to get the parent's attention. Adults from this type of attachment usually use the word "we" instead of "I" in talking about themselves. They can appear bossy and controlling, and they struggle to handle rules. They are full of drama and have the potential to stir the pot. They are often self-sabotaging. These individuals are most likely stuck or overly focused on traumatic events from the past (Cochrane, 2003).

This template can be formed when one parent is rigid and dismissive, while the other is dependent and passive. Sometimes the attachment comes from the primary caregiver being married to an addict. It can also be formed by experiencing covert and/or overt abuse.

The person with ambivalent attachment acts in extremes. He or she maintains a sense of entitlement, exhibiting extremely demanding behavior and a high degree of neediness, or acting with extreme helplessness and being overly submissive, overly indecisive, and overly compliant.

Both extremes are ways to attempt to obtain and guarantee secure attachment with the object of the individual's affection.

However, these behaviors actually cause others to withdraw. And if the person's sense of security is threatened, or there is going to be a separation, extreme behaviors are triggered. "I love you completely and totally. I will do anything to get you to love me. If I think you will leave me, I will hate you just as much as I used to love you."

The problem is that those with an ambivalent attachment template often see themselves as being rejected. As such, there is always a great deal of passion the person's life—passionately loving and passionately hating.

The Ambivalent Attachment Style

Individuals with an ambivalent attachment will tend to:

- Be flooded by distressing emotions and become clingy
- Have heightened emotional expression and vigilance for parental attention
- Try to be intensely involved in others' traumatic pasts
- Feel highly worried about parents' welfare
- Rely on emotional coping rather than cognitive problem-solving
- Have trouble seeing the difference between their own internal view of the world (fear based) and the reality of their situation
- Overestimate severity of dangers and underestimate their own resources
- Be passive and helpless
- Feel overly concerned with trying to please their parents
- Have an inability to handle imperfections in self or others
- Receive a diagnosis of chronic PTSD, with symptoms being particularly intrusive and disruptive in the person's life (Goldberg, 2000)

A person with this type of attachment will have a hard time integrating past and present experiences. He or she finds it difficult to learn from the past and struggles to see his or her ongoing pattern of behavior. The person will make the same mistake over and over again with little or no awareness of the repetitive pattern.

Spiritually, the ambivalent adult will struggle with two faces. One is the face of deep concern for others—he or she is compassionate to a fault, always willing and wanting to help. However, the ambivalent person often gets overly involved in others' problems. Drama always seems to follow this individual, who is a worry wart. The person struggles with faith because he or she is so focused on what's going wrong and how large the problem is. Fear and insecurity and anxiety are bigger than God.

The other face is more hidden—that of being judgmental and critical of oneself and others. As the individual is helping someone, he or she can get angry when that person isn't getting better or following his or her advice. Often an individual with ambivalent attachment has a negative, detrimental running commentary in his or her head about himself or herself. He or she sees himself or herself as beyond the help of the Savior's Atonement. The person wants to believe good works will tip the scales of justice in his or her favor on Judgment Day. Therefore, this individual tries harder to fix, save, help, and redeem others. The person becomes more invested in change than in those he or she is helping.

As with other attachment styles, the ambivalent adult struggles with perfectionism, but he or she will have a more hopeless attitude about it. "I have to be perfectly obedient before God so I can get into heaven, but I never will be." Then they participate in self-destructive behavior as a form of punishment for not being strictly obedient. Essentially, this pattern of thought is all about how bad they are. They become stuck and fixated on how bad they are and seem to forget that the Atonement is waiting for them. Their preoccupation with their own imperfections negates and denies the power of the Christ's ultimate sacrifice.

The Spiritually Ambivalent Attachment Style

People with a spiritually ambivalent attachment style have a tendency to:

- Believe they can "make" God love them or "make" Him hate them; can't trust or believe that God, by Himself, will choose to love them
- Struggle with pride and see themselves as better than others in the congregation by way of spiritual works or scriptural knowledge
- Confuse humility with self-hatred, and godly sorrow with self-pity
- See themselves, in moments of honesty, as wishy-washy when it comes to gospel commitment, and then they punish themselves for not being more committed, which often leads to sin that validates their sense of being beyond the Atonement
- Be open about their problems, but stay stuck in a "woe is me" perspective
- Either see the Atonement as unreachable and as reserved for those who are already holy, or see their sins as so bad that the Savior's sacrifice can't help them
- Possess a spirituality so intense or zealous that it puts others off

What needs to happen spiritually for individuals who have an ambivalent attachment is to calm down, to let go of control, and let God take over. They need to focus on developing faith and hope, and on having a broken heart and contrite spirit. Staying out of others' drama is key. Focusing on anonymous service is a good way to begin. There needs to be a lot of work on positive self-talk. Understanding various concepts of the Atonement, such as grace, justice, mercy, and Heavenly Father's love, will be integral to overcoming this attachment style and be healed.

Case Story

Rex and I worked together for several years. He came from an incestuous family. His mother was a very dominant figure in his life. She was cold and rigid, and she was a perfectionist. He often described her as a supermom. "I can remember listening to her vacuuming at 2:00 AM because guests were coming the next day."

Rex's father was a very intimidating figure until Rex became a teenager. By the time Rex was thirteen years old, his father was opening up and acting very vulnerable with Rex. As an adult, Rex came to see how his father was using him to meet his emotional needs. As an adolescent, Rex described himself as his dad's substitute wife. This made him feel very special, and at the same time, even more lonely. Nobody was there to meet Rex's needs. He had no one to talk to. He had to be there for his dad, and his mother was too judgmental.

When Rex got married, he often had arguments with his wife about his unusual connection to his parents. He felt a strong need to continue to be there for his dad, even at the expense of his relationship with his wife. Rex went out of his way to try to impress his mother. Whenever his parents were going to visit, he would clean the house with an intensity that caused arguments. Now he was the one vacuuming at 2:00 AM.

In therapy, Rex explained how he both hated and loved his parents. He still chased after that feeling of "specialness," and if he couldn't get it from his parents, he started trying to find it with other women. It took him years to realize he was a sex addict. He truly had to struggle to become aware of his patterns of behavior. I often gave him writing assignments to help him in his quest for awareness. This comes from one of his writing exercises, with his permission.

One night, after going to a twelve-step meeting for sex and love addicts, it hit me. All of the people I had become intensely drawn to had themselves been abused in some way during the same period I had. What was almost supernatural was that I never knew of the other person's abuse history until after the intrigue of the relationship had begun.

I believe I was attracted to the covert energy or vibes the other person was giving off. If I were in a room with a bunch of different people, I'd be drawn to these damaged, hurt people who were trying to pretend their abusive childhood wasn't affecting them. There might be others who had an abusive childhood, but if they were in the process of healing, there was no charge of electricity, no vibe of energy, no spark of intensity between us.

What was I hoping for? Why was I drawn to women who were so much like me—disconnected from themselves and hurting inside? The response to this question was earth shattering. It came to me in a flash of awareness around 2:00 AM *one night. My mind suddenly fit more pieces of the puzzle together and I couldn't get back to sleep. I was so excited. I could actually make sense and understand something that had been so hidden and subconscious in its origins for so many years. I was looking for people to play out my childhood with. Either I was the love-obsessed, dependent victim in the scenario (my father), or I was the manipulative and seductive one (my mother). Most of the time I'd switch from one role to the other.*

In terms of his relationship with the Savior, Rex routinely described himself as the exception to the Atonement. "There is no way I can be forgiven," he would lament. Instead of humbling himself, Rex became even more zealous with his priesthood duties. He was the guy who was always there, always helping and always signing up for service projects. Yet after a period of time, he'd crash and almost become inactive. His inability to maintain such a level of service left him feeling worthless. There was no way God was going to wipe away his sins now.

As important as service is, Rex needed to learn some basic gospel principles first. He needed to learn that humility and godly sorrow are not the equivalent of beating himself and hating himself. He needed to learn that a contrite spirit is not the same as self-pity or a "woe is me" mentality. And most importantly, Rex needed to learn that good works without repentance won't make him eligible to return to God's presence.

CHAPTER 12

DISORGANIZED ATTACHMENT

The last major category is disorganized adults. Around 15% to 20% of children experience a disorganized attachment to their primary caregiver. These individuals were raised in homes of serious abuse, neglect, or severe loss. The parents were usually the perpetrators of the abuse. Disorganized attachment is considered to be an extreme form of the avoidant attachment style.

The Disorganized Attachment Style

Individuals who have experienced a disorganized attachment are prone to:

- See themselves as bad, worthless, and undeserving of love
- Be prone to rage
- Dissociate (more so than other attachment types)
- Have a mental health diagnosis of conduct disorder and / or suffer from chronic PTSD
- (As a child) Take responsibility for control within family relationships
- Be controlling and coercive
- Dominate the caregiver either by rejecting or humiliating the parent or by being overly attentive and protective to the parent

- Struggle to move beyond themselves—have difficulty showing compassion or empathy for others
- Act impulsively
- Refuse personal responsibility for their actions; seen as selfish, egocentric, and narcissistic (Stoufe, et al. 2000)

This attachment style is most often caused by hands-on abuse—physical or sexual. Shirley Glass (2003) describes individuals with disorganized attachment as people who don't open up, who don't ponder much about relationships, and who are prone to have one-night stands and multiple affairs. All in all, such individuals are extremely reluctant to make a commitment. They see their partners as being too intrusive and smothering.

The disorganized template sounds something like this: "My walls are to keep me safe. I will never let anyone in, for to do so will cause me to give up my protection from harm. I will do whatever it takes to make sure I am safe." More than anything, safety is paramount—more so than receiving love. People with this attachment style tend to suffer from dissociation more than do those with any other attachment style (Steele, Hart & Nijenhuis, 2001).

The disorganized adult will struggle to connect with past experiences. If he or she moves away, it is difficult for him or her to maintain friendships. If the other person isn't right there in front of the disorganized adult, it is as though the friendship doesn't exist. If the disorganized person served a mission, it will seem like a faraway dream. This individual has learned how to put on a mask and can be superficially charming. His or her internal life, and thus his or her testimony, appears strong until tested. With a trial or a life challenge, that testimony quickly fades and the person's faith flounders.

The opposite is also true. Instead of still trying to maintain a connection with God and the Church, the disorganized adult can be angry, hostile, or at the very least, passive in his or her relationship to God. The person will struggle with the basic belief that Heavenly Father is always there, always loving, and always listening. A disorganized adult will often attend church because of a parent or a spouse, rather than due to his or her own personal testimony.

The Spiritually Disorganized Attachment Style

Individuals with a spiritually disorganized attachment have a tendency to:

- Struggle with the basic concept of faith; may be skeptical about God's existence
- Doubt that Christ understands what they have gone through; feel cynical about His ability to heal them or forgive them
- Get stuck wondering how God could love them and yet allow them to be abused
- Attend church at the urging of others (such as a spouse, parent, or close friend)
- Struggle to feel the Spirit, not necessarily because of sin but because they are so cut off from their emotions
- See others' tenderness or sensitivity as a sign of weakness
- Struggle with being humble and teachable; see the commandments as a form of control and domination—as chains that keep them from "true freedom"
- Feel exposed if they do open up or feel God's love; this brings a knee-jerk reaction to withdraw from others
- Believe having a broken heart and a contrite spirit is a sign of weakness; see vulnerability as the worst possible thing someone could feel or experience

To overcome this attachment style and truly connect to the Savior and His Atonement, the person must develop an internal connection with himself or herself. Because he or she dissociates so much—disconnecting from emotions, internal sensations, and life experiences—there is an absolute need for the individual to own his or her life. The person needs to plug back into the physical and emotional network between the mind and heart, the brain and body. Creating a safe environment is essential to help facilitate this reawakening. And when love is felt, it is critical to sit with the experience and not run away from it. Over time, feeling God's love will be seen as safe and nurturing. Then, the door can be opened to experience the healing and restorative powers of the Atonement.

Case Story

Lisa endured terrible abuse in her childhood. She joined the Church in her early thirties. It was not an easy fit for her. She longed for the sweet feelings of peace from the Holy Ghost, but struggled to stay in a place where she could have those experiences. Lisa routinely commented how the word "vulnerable" was a terrible word, and she even screwed up her face like she was eating something disgusting whenever we talked about opening up.

Feeling anything was hard for Lisa. Most of the time she was in her head. Whenever I asked her what she was experiencing in her body, she would shrug and say, "Nothing. It's blank in there. I don't feel anything."

At times she would call and have me come over to dump out bottles of alcohol or throw away bags of meth. Whatever she had to do to stay away from the past, she would try. The ironic thing was, the harder she tried to run away from the past, the harder it was for her to stay in the present.

Eventually Lisa agreed to stop running. We discussed how facing the past isn't about reliving it. Facing the past is about acknowledging it and eventually owning it. It is seeing how the past affects our present thoughts, attitudes, and beliefs. There is no need to submerge ourselves in the terror of the past, but there is a need to let the story of our past be told. This kind of work is all about seeking to become whole, not fragmented.

Spiritually, Lisa wanted to control everything. And not being able to control things when it came to the Atonement frustrated her to no end. "I hate it when you talk about God's timing! I'm ready now! Why wouldn't He want me to feel free of my past? Why would He want me to stay in this pain?"

"Maybe because the day-to-day process you are going through is actually essential to your growth and healing," I suggested.

"But you tell me to pray for comfort, and it doesn't come! You tell me Heavenly Father is there, but I don't feel Him."

I nodded my head. I understood her frustration. "Lisa, the very thing you need to experience—love—has become your worst fear. You are so afraid of feeling love that you run from it. Love requires that you be open to it and accept it. You have to let down your walls for God to touch your heart. You pray for healing and comfort, but you don't want to open up for that to happen."

"Can't He do it with the door locked—like slide it under the door?" Lisa asked with a sad smile on her face. "Maybe He can leave it outside, ring the doorbell and then leave . . ."

I laughed. "God's love is not like a UPS package. And let's not forget it's the abuse that tainted your views about love and about being open to love. It is a logical and biological reaction to the extreme trauma you experienced. But as I've said before, that was then and this is now. We need to help your brain and body understand that you are not in danger right now. You don't need to keep being in survival mode. You don't need to keep dissociating and looking for a way to escape. And most importantly, God's love doesn't hurt."

Lisa sighed and flopped her arms down on the couch in resignation. "I know, but staying in reality is really hard. Everything still sets me off. I don't know how to not react like I'm in danger."

"Well, let's work on that."

What I taught Lisa and others is that so much of our self-talk reinforces old messages and beliefs that are twisted and distorted. It's hard to make changes when there is a steady, negative chatter inside your head about how bad and worthless you are. To counter all that negative self-talk, there is a need to affirm yourself. I often rolled my eyes at people who did positive affirmations until I started doing my own work. What I found was that there is great power in giving myself a positive affirmation. It didn't heal me, but it did open me up to change.

Affirmations for Overcoming Arrested Developmental Stages

The following affirmations are excerpts from the book *Growing Up Again*. Pick one that corresponds with the age when your trauma occurred. Repeat it a hundred times a day, in one sitting. After a couple of months, pick another one. Maybe you will read the list and feel drawn to a particular statement. It may have nothing to do with when you were abused, but nevertheless it is a message some part of you needs to hear.

Conception to Birth

- "I celebrate that you are alive."
- "I love you just as you are."

Birth to Six Months

- "What you need is important to me."
- "I love you and I care for you willingly."
- "You can grow at your own pace."

Six Months to Eighteen Months

- "You can explore and experiment, and I will support and protect you."
- "You can do things as many times as you need to in order to learn and grow."

Eighteen Months to Three Years

- "It's okay for you to be angry, and I will provide boundaries so you won't feel out of control with your anger."
- "You can say no and push and test limits as much as you need to."
- "You can become separate from me and I will continue to love you."

Three Years to Six Years

- "You can be powerful and ask for help at the same time."
- "All of your feelings are okay with me."
- "I love who you are and who you are becoming."

Six Years to Twelve Years

- "You can think before you say yes or no and learn from your mistakes."
- "You can trust your intuition to help you decide what to do."
- "I love you even when we differ; I love growing with you."

Part 3

Building Faith

Strengthen ye the weak hands, and confirm the feeble knees. Say to them that are of a fearful heart, Be strong, fear not: behold your God will come with vengeance, even God with a recompence; he will come and save you. Then the eyes of the blind shall be opened, and the ears of the deaf shall be unstopped. —Isaiah 35:3–5

Chapter 13
Session with Terri

Taking in the physical damage of Terri's soul-stretching fight, I observed, "You look terrible."

"Yeah, well I'm not trying to hide it anymore. No more putting on a mask, screwing on some stupid smile, and telling everyone that everything is fine."

"Good. You are being true to yourself. We call that being congruent. It's where your insides match your outsides—no more fake."

"Unfortunately, I'm afraid I'm going to have to drop out of the Miss America pageant."

I laughed, which brought a small smile to her face.

There was a lull in the conversation. I waited, watching while she curled up even more on the couch as though she wanted the cushions to swallow her.

"You don't like it when I ask you to untangle yourself and take in a deep breath, do you?" I said finally.

Terri rolled her eyes. "Oh no. You are always asking me to uncross my arms and legs. You are always trying to get me to breathe and open up. You should know by now that I don't do open."

"Why is that?"

"Uh, Mr. Therapist, you're asking a question I know you know the answer to."

I acknowledged her statement with a nod. "Humor me."

"I don't do open like I don't do vulnerable."

"Because . . ."

"Because being open makes bad things happen."

"Like what?"

"Like feeling stuff. Like remembering stuff. Like experiencing stuff."

"Isn't that what we're here to do—to feel, to acknowledge, and to accept?"

"No. You have to help me find a way to heal without feeling."

I laughed. "Everyone tries to find that way. It doesn't exist."

"Why not?" Terri put on a little show of pouting. "It's not fair."

"You're right, it isn't. The way to heal is through the body, and the body is usually the last place we want to connect to."

"That's true. I hate my body."

"You mean you don't like the way it looks?"

"No, I mean I hate what's *in* my body. Pain is in my body. Memories are in my body. Terrible icky and gross and disgusting sludge is in my body. I try every day not to be in my body. It's the last place I want to be."

"Isn't it interesting that the adversary, who will never have a body, works so hard to get us to hate our bodies," I thought out loud.

"How can I not hate it?" Terri went on. "I am constantly reminded of what happened to me. I can't escape it because it's—" she pointed to herself "—it's in there."

"What's in there?"

She clenched her teeth. "The grossness."

"What is the grossness like?"

Terri wiped her hands as if she was washing them. Her face took on a disgusted look. "The grossness of the abuse—it's like tar, or black sludge."

"Where is it in your body?" I asked. She pointed to her stomach and to her arms. "What does it look like in your stomach?"

"It's like a ball, sitting in the very center of me."

"What's it like to feel that heavy-sludge grossness in the very center of you?"

Terri closed her eyes and held her stomach with both hands. "It makes me feel heavy and slow and tired."

"Like you want to go to sleep?" I said. She nodded. "Okay, I want you to stand up, Terri."

"Why?" she whined.

"Because when you want to go to sleep like this, you are dissociating. There is no healing in disappearing. So stand up."

Reluctantly, and with great protest, she stood up.

"Good. Now I want you to push your feet into the floor. Yes, that's right. And I want you to keep your hands on your tummy. Is that heavy sludge ball still there?"

She nodded. "Yeah, and I think I'm gonna throw up."

I brought out my garbage can. "That's okay if you have to."

"Can I sit down now?"

"No. What does that gross ball in your gut say? What would it say if it could speak?"

Without a pause, Terri responded, "It would swear and cuss and say that I'm a loser."

"A loser? Why?"

"Because it's all my fault! The abuse was all my fault! And what kind of a sick, twisted little girl am I to want these things to happen to me?" She fell back into the couch and hid her face from me as she burrowed into the couch pillows. "I'm gross and disgusting! It's me! I am!"

"I thought you had this icky sludge ball inside of you that was gross and disgusting. I thought that was disgusting, not you."

"No, it's me. I am!" she yelled, her voice muffled by the pillows.

I waited quietly. Eventually she sat up and rubbed tears from her eyes. Very softly, I began to talk. "Terri, what just happened is that you went from *feeling* an emotion to *becoming* an emotion. You were connecting to feelings about the abuse. Then you became the feelings about the abuse. This is how we get stuck. This is why we run away from our bodies. This is why we often say things like 'My pain is bigger than me,' or 'my fear swallowed me up.' We become the emotion, instead of simply experiencing it."

"But I feel disgusted."

"Yes, but that is different than *being* disgusting."

"But I feel gross." She wiped her arms in a downward motion. "It's like I can feel the gross sludge on my skin." She shook her hands like she was trying to get the sludge off of her fingers.

"Yes, you *feel* gross, but you are not gross." I handed her a towel. "Here, take this and wipe away the sludge."

Terri gave me a funny look, but I persisted. As she started to wipe down one arm, and then the other, her skeptical, self-conscious attitude disappeared. "And what about your legs?" I said. With great conviction, she began to vigorously wipe down her legs. "Don't forget your face," I urged. She responded by wiping her face, and then her head and neck.

"Do you need another towel?" I asked. She nodded. I gave her another one. She wiped around her belly, her back, and her feet. Watching her do this, it was very clear to me that she actually felt something slimy and gunky on her. It was invisible, but yet very real. And this ritual cleansing seemed to have an effect on her. She began muttering to herself.

"Say it out loud," I encouraged.

"You will never touch my body again," she said with great force as she wiped her leg again. I gave her another towel. She took it, and as she wiped her arms again, she repeatedly said, "You will never touch my body again."

When it was over, I had five towels in a heap on the floor.

"How do you feel?" I asked.

Terri took a deep breath. It took her a minute to answer. "I feel . . . lighter."

"What was this experience like for you?"

She shook her head in disbelief. "At first I thought you were crazy, but as I wiped the towel down my arm, I felt something. It felt real. Then suddenly all I wanted to do was wipe this sludge off of me. It was everywhere, and I couldn't use the towel fast enough. It kept gushing out. And I had to keep wiping it away."

"That's great. You unloaded some of that trapped grossness from the abuse. But we're not quite done yet. I want you to recheck—to take a look inside and see if that ball is still there."

Terri closed her eyes. "If it is there, it's really small."

"Good. Okay, now in the space that was once filled with this grossness, we want to invite love in. We want sunshine to come in and fill those empty spaces. We want God to come in and fill those places with His love."

"How do I do that?" Terri murmured.

"I want you to tell Heavenly Father what just happened and ask Him to fill your empty spaces with His love."

"Right now?"

"Yes."

"God, I just got rid of a bunch of slimy gunk," she began. "It was all this black sludge from when I was sexually abused. It just came pouring out of me. I feel like there is this physical space inside of me now. It's really weird how real it feels. I don't want this empty space to be filled back up with this icky stuff." Terri's voice broke, and she started to cry. "I don't ever want that back!" she cried out. "Please fill these empty spaces with Thy love. Please." She suddenly became very quiet and then started crying again, but this time she had a smile on her face.

"What happened?" I asked quietly.

She looked at me and smiled. "I felt it."

"Felt what?"

"I felt His love. It was like this warm light, and I was wrapped up in it, and it filled me from the bottom of my feet to the top of my head."

I smiled back at her. I had just witnessed a miracle. This woman who had previously said she couldn't feel God's love, let alone anything else, had suddenly made a real connection to Heaven. She experienced Heavenly Father's love and knew for the first time that it was safe to be open. Love could be healing. Love from a man could be safe. This wasn't the end of her journey, but it was a pivotal moment.

Chapter 14
A Crumbling Foundation

The Atonement of Jesus Christ is a miracle and a wonder. It has the power to wash us clean. It can comfort us and give us hope. It can heal broken hearts and wounded minds. The Atonement can empower us, through grace, giving us strength beyond our own. It fuels change. It is the power of change. Through the Atonement, we can rise above the destructive and limiting patterns from our past. Our brains can be rewired and we can receive new hearts, opening the doors to a new way of thinking, feeling, and living. In the Old Testament, the Lord declared, "A new heart also will I give you, and a new spirit will I put within you: and I will take away the stony heart out of your flesh, and I will give you an heart of flesh" (Ezekiel 36:26).

The first step in accessing this transformative power is faith. Elder Richard G. Scott stated: "Remember an unfailing, continual, ever-present source of peace and comfort is available to you. It is the certainty that your Father in Heaven loves you no matter what your circumstance, no matter what winds of trial, turmoil, or tribulation whirl about you. That certainty will never change. *Your ability to access that support depends on the strength of your faith in Him* and in His certain willingness to bless you" (Scott, 2003; italics added).

My wife and I love watching the cable channel HGTV, where houses get renovated or restored. Sometimes the houses people buy end up having foundation issues—a problem that has not been budgeted in the renovation. There is a crack, or parts are crumbling, or the wood is rotted. In one episode of *Rehab Addict,* the host had to literally jack up the house and put in a new foundation.

I love seeing dilapidated or really ugly houses get a second chance. It is as if new life is breathed into the structure. The process is rough, and often the homeowners can't hold the vision that the hosts and crew have as they tear down, dismantle, and even destroy parts of the home. At the end, when the reveal takes place and the workmen give the homeowners a tour of the "new" house, it is always breathtaking. The owners cry with joy and talk about how they had trouble believing and trusting the hosts that their home would come through all the renovation chaos.

So it is with overcoming childhood abuse. Our lives are the broken, abandoned houses. Heavenly Father shows us how He can restore us and even make our lives better. The process is rough, sometimes excruciatingly painful. Yet God continually reminds us that He can see the beginning from the end. He knows what needs to happen. President Dieter F. Uchtdorf declared: "The Lord said to Abraham, 'My name is Jehovah, and I know the end from the beginning; therefore my hand shall be over thee' (Abr. 2:8) . . . today I say to you that if you trust the Lord and obey Him, His hand shall be over you, He will help you achieve the great potential He sees in you, and He will help you to see the end from the beginning" (Uchtdorf, 2006).

The problem is, we often don't trust the Lord with our lives. When there was no one else to help us, we tried to hold up our crumbling foundation ourselves. When there was no safe place, we relied on ourselves to create safety. When we had no way to manage the pain and fear, we found ways to escape.

Nothing destroys faith as quickly and completely as abuse. It overwhelms us with fear, terror, and confusion. It creates beliefs that breed future doubts. It sows seeds of anger, resentments, and even rage. Yes, abuse has the power to build walls against anyone or anything that might eventually help, support, and even heal the wounded individual. How, therefore, can we create, build, and foster faith when abuse usually happens while our very foundations are being poured and built? The answer is not pretty. For most of us who suffered childhood abuse, our emotional, mental, and spiritual foundations are full of cracks, crumbling concrete, and rotten wood. Faith is built on a shaky foundation, making it weak and unsteady.

A basic belief many people adopt from experiencing physical, verbal, or sexual abuse is that trusting someone is what caused us to get hurt in the first place. That is a lie, but one that is so easy to believe. Even if we knew exactly what was going to happen, and knew the true intentions of our abusers, the reality is that we were children, and no amount of knowledge of the future could save us. We were powerless. And nobody likes to feel powerless.

We tell ourselves that if we had known hidden motivations, if we hadn't been so naive, if we hadn't trusted this person or that person, we would have been safe and the abuse would have never happened. That idea creates a possibility that maybe we could have power over future abuse.

As we try to turn to the Savior and use His Atonement to comfort and heal us, He asks us to do the very thing we believed got us into trouble in the first place—trust Him and have faith in Him. President Henry B. Eyring stated, "God . . . loves us and wants our happiness. And He knows how a lack of trust in Him brings sadness" (Eyring, 2010). How on earth can we break the chains of our traumatic past and feel the peace we have so desperately dreamed of, if we cannot trust God? We are left with a deep and profound sadness, a heaviness that weighs us down in despair and misery. For many of us, we feel stuck—damned if we do open up, and damned if we don't open up.

Case Story

Dennis came to see me on a sunny morning. He was nervous and appeared agitated. He was addicted to pornography, but on this day, we were going to talk about some of the underlying issues in his life. He was nervous because he claimed he didn't like talking about his past.

"I notice you keep your hair very short. Were you in the military?" I asked.

He shook his head. "Nah, I just like my hair short."

"Oh, okay. It's just that most people don't go that short."

"I don't like long hair."

"Why not?"

"It's no big deal. Let's talk about something else."

I smiled and gave a little laugh. "You do realize that if you say something like that to a therapist, that is exactly what ends up being talked about."

"I don't like long hair because—because my dad used to grab my hair and march me around the house, showing me all the messes I'd made. I could barely keep up with him. I had to walk on my tippy toes to alleviate some of the pain in my scalp."

"How old were you when this happened?"

"I dunno, maybe six or seven," Dennis replied. "He kept doin' it until I was ten or so."

"So you keep very short hair so that you father can't pull your hair anymore?"

"Hey, nobody is going to yank on my hair ever again. Do you know that he actually detached my scalp from the back part of my skull in some places? I don't have any feeling back here." Dennis pointed to the back of his head.

"Wow."

"Yeah, wow is right."

"Sounds like your dad was pretty abusive."

"He was a real stickler for having everything in its place."

"He sounds very rigid and controlling," I commented. Dennis nodded his head. I thought for a moment and then asked him, "Do you have trouble with authority figures?"

"Like who?"

"Police, bosses, Church leaders . . . maybe even God."

Dennis gave a short laugh. "God has had it in for me as long as I can remember. I've always been a disappointment to Him."

"Oh? How do you know that?"

"Remember why I'm here? I'm a member of His Church and I can't stop looking at porn! Of course He's upset with me."

"Maybe He wants to pull your hair too," I quietly suggested.

Dennis grinned a little. "I don't doubt it."

"Did you ever stop to think that maybe how you see and interpret God's attitude toward you has been shaped by the past experiences you had with your father?"

"What?"

"Or to put it another way, God is not your dad."

"I know that," Dennis snorted.

"Do you? Look at the way you think God is going to react to your porn addiction. It sounds like He is without mercy, love or compassion. It sounds like He expects you to stop but He isn't going to give you any guidance. Does that sound like anyone you know?"

Dennis thought, his eyebrows crunching up. He sat back in his chair and took a breath. "You think I confuse God with my father."

I nodded.

"But God hates sinners," Dennis declared. "He's always blasting them off the face of the earth!"

I lifted my finger. "Ah, but you're forgetting something. The Lord only does that to those who aren't repenting after they had chance after chance to do so."

"But I keep messing up."

"And do you keep picking yourself back up and try again?"

"Yeah."

"Then you don't fall into that other category of sinners, do you?"

"I guess not," Dennis said.

"And God does love the sinners. It's the sin He can't tolerate."

"But I always feel so bad when I fall down. I get scared."

"Of what?"

"Of God losing His temper with me."

"Oh . . . that sounds like something you worried about when you were a little boy and your dad got angry about something."

Dennis nodded his head.

"It must be hard to trust God when you are afraid of Him."

Dennis nodded again and looked down at the floor. "Everyone talks about the power of the Atonement, how it can heal and cleanse and help us repent, but I've never felt that."

"It's pretty hard to access the Atonement when you are afraid of God," I said. "Fear and faith are like magnets—they repel each other. It's hard to hold onto faith when we're full of fear."

"I guess I'm screwed then. I can't have faith, even though that is exactly what I need to get better."

I held up my hands. "Whoa. Who said anything about not being able to have faith? You can and will. We just need to separate your dad from God. We need to learn who God really is. Joseph Smith said we can't have faith in God if we don't know who He is or what He is like. Let's find out how Heavenly Father is different than your earthly father."

Over time, Dennis learned to exercise faith in Heavenly Father. He had to divorce his image of his mortal father from God's image. Once that happened, Dennis could make a sincere connection with Heavenly Father. He came to feel love and support from God. He realized God wasn't ever going to hurt him or "pull his hair."

Dennis's story reminds us that faith can be corroded when we have an incorrect idea of who God is, when we struggle with low self-esteem, when we block our emotions, and when we feel paralyzed with fear. These belief-stealing variables are common side effects of abuse. It is devilish intelligence to create a sin that can continue to be felt for decades after the act has been committed. For Satan, it's not enough to get someone to sin once. He wants that sin to affect as many people as possible for as long as possible. And since faith is a necessary ingredient to accessing the Atonement and healing from the past, it is what the devil targets as often as he can.

Part of what makes having faith in God hard is that we have experienced a godlike person in our lives already and nothing good came from it. Our abusers were godlike. During the abuse, there was no option to say no. And if they were our parents, we were forced to interact with and trust these most untrustworthy people with our lives. This definitely will shade and twist the notion that God can be trusted.

We have to reconnect to God. We have to relearn who He is and what His personality is like. We have to throw away all our outdated and false ideas about Him. That takes time. But the Holy Ghost will help us immensely in this area. He will help us to see that our deeply held, perhaps even hidden beliefs about God were incorrect. He will help us to discover the difference between our distorted beliefs and the actual truth. We must divorce our abusers completely from who God is and how He feels about us. Then faith can grow.

In the following chapters, let's look in greater detail at three of the greatest variables that are linked to nearly every stumbling block and every maladaptive coping skill that abuse breeds: low self-esteem, blocking emotions, and fear. Sessions with Barry, Rex, and Lisa will show the struggle one can have when these variables are at play and how to overcome them.

Remember, faith is the key that unlocks the power of the Atonement. Without it there is no hope for change, no hope for healing, and no hope for freedom from the past. We will remain victims of the past, prisoners of our childhood pain. We must do all we can find faith in Heavenly Father and in His Son, Jesus Christ.

As we explore how we can do that, hold fast. Changes don't happen overnight. As your faith grows, hold fast. As it is strengthened and nurtured, hold fast. As your faith becomes stronger than your fears, hold fast. There may be moments where nothing makes sense, where you can't see the end of the journey, where you feel stuck and bogged down in the gunky, mucky parts of your past. In those moments, hold fast.

CHAPTER 15

SELF-ESTEEM

A person with low self-esteem sees his or her relationship with self, with others, and with God through a twisted filter. Since self-esteem is the degree to which an individual believes he or she has worth and value, it is a belief he or she can influence. For instance, if Tara sees herself as terrible, unlovable, and worthless, she will tend to believe that God will not help her, or that even if He could, He wouldn't want to. It is easy to see, then, how faith is negatively impacted by low self-esteem.

From this doubting place, questions like these are asked:

- How can I trust Christ when He says He'll carry my burdens if I yoke myself to Him? I trusted my mother or father or my uncle, and terrible things happened.
- How can I believe that Heavenly Father wants to save me if I am such a disappointment?
- How could anyone, let alone God, love me if they knew who I really was, or if they found out what happened to me?

Faith is built on truth. Yet for most traumatized children, their concept of who they are is impacted by the abuse. It is easy to see how these beliefs are distorted and twisted. The conclusions such individuals draw are based on the information they have at that moment. So, believing I am stupid and a bad son because my father hits me, or that I am unlovable because my mother yells at me all the time, become easy to accept as truth. There is very little good ground for planting seeds of self-confidence or allowing God's love to have a place to grow in my frightened heart. The following are a few lies we tell ourselves when we have low self-esteem:

- I am worthless and awful and no good.
- I am beyond God's help.
- Heavenly Father or Jesus Christ or the Holy Ghost are unreliable and untrustworthy.
- My imperfections, character weaknesses, and sins make God love me less.
- Being perfectly obedient can somehow increase my worth and value.

If these lies were true, it would mean we could make God love us or hate us, that we had the power to change His mind. It would also mean we could create exceptions to rules and eternal laws.

Faith requires truth. The truth is that regardless of what has happened to us or how the past has influenced our poor choices, God is the Father of our spirits and He loves us with an eternal and endless love. Nothing can ever change that.

Case Story

Barry's eyes were full of fire. "I am surrounded by ungrateful, selfish, and stupid people. So I looked at a little porn, so maybe I flirt with the waitress a little. So maybe I had a couple of slip-ups and made out with some coworkers at that conference down in Los Angeles. What do you think they would do if I stopped paying for everything?"

"I don't think you're in much of a position to compare your sexual addiction to their ingratitude," I said. "Besides, money isn't the issue."

"It wasn't like I had sex with anyone. I didn't hurt anyone."

I raised my eyebrows and started to interrupt, but Barry was on a roll. I knew what he wanted me to do. We had been here plenty of times before. He wanted to vent and say everything he couldn't say to his wife or bishop, without me interrupting and correcting his twisted perspective.

"I demand respect," Barry went on. "They can't just walk all over me and make demands. They need to show gratitude for the money I bring home!"

"This isn't the issue."

"Let's see how they act when I stop paying for their cell phones and car insurance and drop them from my health insurance."

"This isn't the issue," I repeated.

Barry rambled on for nearly ten minutes, swearing and cursing his wife and children for how disrespectful they were toward him, how unfairly and unjustly he was being treated.

"Barry!" I yelled. That got his attention. "Money is not the issue. Your children's ingratitude isn't the issue."

"But—"

"No," I interrupted. "Listen." I held up one hand and cupped it. "Here you have Barry the sex addict. He is a worthless piece of trash. He is, quoting you, a disgusting pervert." I lifted my other hand and cupped it. "Over here, is Barry the 'Great Provider.' He is hailed by all at work as one of the best in the company. He gets raises and emails from his bosses and supervisors, extolling his virtues."

"And which Barry do your wife and children focus on? Barry the pervert or Barry the successful breadwinner?"

"Barry the pervert," he said angrily.

"Right. And how does that make you feel?"

"Lousy! Can't they—"

I interrupted again. "Nope, wait. This has nothing to do with their ingratitude. You just don't want to see the fact that Barry the sex addict has lost all credibility with his family. You want them to recognize your hard work and the successful part of your life. Then maybe you will feel better about yourself."

"I pay for their—"

"Barry! No, it's not about the money. You don't like seeing yourself as—how did you say it? A worthless pervert?"

He stopped talking and barely nodded.

"This isn't about anyone else—what they did or didn't do, how they may have slighted you, or how disrespectful someone may be toward you. This is about how you see yourself. Self-esteem is the degree to which we believe we have worth and value. So, based on your belief, your worth and value can go up or down." I paused. "But it is only our belief—our perception—that changes. Actually, our worth and value is unchanging. It is fixed. It is infinite."

Barry shook his head. "No, that can't be right. If I do well in my company, they see me as being a valuable team member and give me a raise. If I do horrible at work, my boss will see me as worthless and fire me."

"Those are consequences based on choices you make at work," I replied. "Your worth and value as a person, as a child of God, cannot diminish or be enlarged."

"This doesn't make any sense. The stake president has more worth than I do. He is the stake president."

"No, Barry. He doesn't have more worth than you do."

"What? Of course he does. He is more righteous than I am. The Lord can use him as an instrument to help lots of people's lives. God can't use me."

"Whether or not God can use you has nothing to do with your worth and value. Your spiritual state of being righteous or being a sinner does not affect your worth and value. Your calling in the Church does not determine your worth and value."

"Of course it does! Look at Alma and Korihor. Alma definitely had more worth and value than Korihor did."

"No, and here's why. Both of those men were sons of God. What gives us worth and value is the fact that God is our spiritual Father. It is the unalterable relationship between God and us that gives us our worth and value."

"And if I am a bad son, I am worthless to God."

I shook my head. "Come on, you know that isn't true. The Lord says He leaves the ninety and nine and goes after the one—the sinner. And what about the prodigal son? Or how about John 3:16–17: 'For God so loved the world, that he gave his only begotten Son, that whosoever believeth in him should not perish, but have everlasting life. For God sent not his Son into the world to condemn the world; but that the world through him might be saved.'"

"Let me make this scripture more personal," I continued. "'For God so loved Barry that He gave His only begotten Son.' See how much God loves you? And this verse implies that you are already in a sinful state. So Heavenly Father is saying, 'Even in the state you are in, I love you. I love you enough to allow my only begotten Son to suffer for your sins so you can home to me.'"

"This doesn't make sense," Barry mumbled.

"You can't make God hate you, and you can't make Him love you. He has already chosen to love you no matter what. You are 100% His son. Can you make yourself 110% His spiritual son? Or how about only 85% His son? Of course not. That's like saying I can physically refuse 40% of the genetic DNA I got from my mother. It's impossible."

"I hear what you are saying, but it still doesn't make sense," Barry said quietly, his anger gone.

"Your worth and value is linked to your relationship with God. And you are 100% His son."

"But He must have favorites," Barry argued.

I shook my head. "No. The stake president is 100% Heavenly Father's son. And so are you and so am I. His worth and value is the same as yours because you are both literally the offspring of God."

"Yes, but look at what the stake president does and look at what I do."

"The stake president makes choices that create consequences, just like you or I do. Sometimes the consequences are good. And when they are, blessings flow to many. And when they aren't good, sadness and pain are often felt."

"So the consequences of my choices determine my worth and value."

"No. Your worth and value is as fixed as your literal connection to Heavenly Father. Your choices and the resulting consequences have nothing to do with that."

"But it sure looks like the righteous are highly favored of the Lord."

"When we are righteous, we receive more blessings from God—that is true. But receiving blessings as a consequence of keeping commandments is not validation of your worth and value. The validation of your worth and value comes in knowing you are God's son. Nothing can ever change that. God does not disown you."

"What happens if I don't make it to the celestial kingdom? I'll be disowned then. That will show my lack of worth and value." Barry was looking more and more confused.

"Nope. Stay with me," I told him. "You've almost got it. Making it to the celestial kingdom has nothing to do with your worth or value. The placement in the afterlife is based on choices you make, not on your worth and value. Nothing can erase who your Eternal Parents are, no matter which degree of glory you inherit."

I stopped talking and waited. In some ways Barry was a very intelligent man, and I was sure his IQ was much higher than mine. Yet his knowledge often became his greatest stumbling block. He could make an argument and appear completely sound and rational, yet that argument contained twisted and distorted truths. He could rationalize and justify and completely believe his own lies. Sometimes this meant I had to be a bit more blunt with him than other clients.

Barry had been horribly abused when he was a child. Unfortunately, it started very early and the older he got, the more severe it became. By the time he was five, most of the damage had been done. His grandfather was often the one who hurt little Barry, but he died when Barry was seven. From then on his parents, with their ongoing abuse, continued to solidify the twisted lies and distorted truths he had learned. It was a miracle Barry could function as well as he did.

As he sat in my office with a faraway look in his eyes, I could see he was processing our discussion. Quietly, he whispered, "This could be a paradigm shift. This could change everything." I nodded. He thought some more. "This is where pride comes in, right?"

"Yes," I said. "Remember that self-esteem is the degree to which we *believe*" —I put a lot of emphasis on that word— "we have worth and value. Our pride can be on a roller coaster just as much as our self-esteem. I can see myself as 'one up' above someone else. And when that person is treated the same way I am, I can become offended. And if I make a mistake, and see myself as 'one down' from someone else, I can be angry at how unfair life is or believe I am beyond hope or love."

I shaped my hand into a hole and peered through it. "See, the adversary will focus on my belief or perception of my worth and value. He will zero in on it and try to manipulate it. He wants you to believe you can get more or lose what you have. Heavenly

Father will also try to influence your belief by reminding you of your relationship to Him."

Barry's eyes got wider. "That's why people say you are a daughter of God or a child of God and He loves you. It is supposed to help us and make us feel better. It is supposed to build us up."

"Uh-huh."

"But it doesn't. Not for me."

"Because you don't believe you have worth and value. Your *belief* about your worth and value is moldable and malleable. Your worth and value isn't. Your focus needs to be on feeling, seeing, and experiencing that relationship with God. Then, when someone reminds you that you are a child of God, it will have an impact on you. It will mean something."

Barry looked exhausted. "I still don't get it."

"So your homework assignment is to review John 3:16 and think about it."

As I walked him out, the Pacific Northwest rain was coming down and there was a slight chill in the air. He put out his hand and I shook it. Smiling, I said, "This was a great session. This really can be the start of that paradigm shift you mentioned."

"Why is it that whenever you say what a great session we had, I leave feeling like I got hit over the head with a two-by-four?" he asked with a sly grin.

"Good sessions are like that. It means you got knocked around enough that maybe some sense got into you." Barry laughed and walked away.

Chapter 16
Blocking Our Emotions

When a person has a traumatic, overpowering experience, the brain tries to find a way to manage the overwhelming incoming data. If the brain can cut up, dissect, and compartmentalize the physical and emotional sensations bombarding the brain and body, there will be a greater chance of survival. If the traumatic events are repeated, the brain quickly learns to adopt these strategies as reactions not only to trauma, but anything that looks like, feels like, smells like, or acts like trauma. The brain remains on high alert.

Over time, emotions—not the actual abuse—become the enemy. Emotions trigger the brain to ramp up our defenses and survival mode. Emotions are the reminders of the abuse. They are the connectors of past memories to the present. Emotions can make us hold our breath, cause our body to stiffen up, or twist our stomach into knots. As Ann Pritt explained in an *Ensign* article: "A basic defense children use against sexual abuse is to shut down their feelings, helping them to get through the trauma. Yet this response also cuts them off from positive feelings. As a result, those who have been sexually abused may have difficulty feeling the love of Heavenly Father, His servants, and other nurturing people in their lives" (Pritt, 2001).

Without emotions, it is difficult to connect to self and others. The result is a deep loneliness. Feelings of betrayal, rejection, and abandonment surface when parents wound a child, whether consciously or not. "I can be in a crowd of people—even surrounded by people I know—and still feel lonely inside," Rex often remarked. Indeed, this sentiment is a common one. Wounded adults fear being alone, based on their damaging experiences as children. Most of us remain stuck in various stages of emotional development, regardless of our physical age. So, in many instances, what drives or pushes us to return over and over again to dysfunctional, maladaptive patterns comes from a frozen, wounded child place within our psyche.

Children fear being left alone—being abandoned—and with good reason. They know they are dependent on others for survival—for food, clothing, and shelter. These basic physical needs are critical, but just as important are children's emotional needs. If a child believes the primary caretaker doesn't like him or her, is overwhelmed with trying to meet his or her needs, or blames the child for the adult's pain and suffering, it is easy for a child to conclude that he or she won't be taken care of. A child learns quickly that the way a person is treated reflects how important that person is to others. If Mommy is depressed, drunk, and always going out with different men (rarely being home or available), the child learns to see himself or herself as not important. Unimportant things get put on a high shelf to be covered in dust and forgotten. That is just as terrifying a thought as it is to think about going hungry. To see a starving child due to the neglect of a parent is heartbreaking. Looking into the eyes of an emotionally wounded child is no less gut-wrenching.

Physical and emotional neglect creates a deficit or lack of feeling loved. This deprivation of love has a significant impact on growth and development. To be deprived of love, validation, support, and nurturing comfort can lead to embracing that type of life and create a state of self-deprivation—denying one's needs and wants.

A client of mine put it bluntly: "If I was a good girl, maybe Mommy and Daddy would notice me." She was described by her parents as the easiest child they had, and in a moment of self-reflective honesty, they said they also believed she was the most neglected of all their children. Being needless and wantless meant she wasn't a burden to her parents, which meant maybe they would love her. Her exact words were "Maybe they will like me then." It is an odd but revealing statement for a child to make about her parents.

Experiencing deprivation as a child is not always remembered as an adult. Severe deprivation, such as being denied sufficient food or clothing, is very stark and obvious, but more subtle forms of deprivation can be just as damaging to a person's psyche. The following are forms of emotional deprivation:

- Touch—lack of physical affection
- Hearing—lack of being heard and acknowledged
- Seeing—lack of supervision, lack of being noticed
- Support—lack of being supported in outside activities, school, grades, etc.
- Basic—lack of adequate food, clothing, or shelter
- Spiritual—lack of validating worth, lack of offering connection to God
- Boundary—lack of teaching, offering, or respecting one's personal space

Deprivation encourages and fosters a profound sense of loneliness. In one session, Rex allowed that little wounded part of him to talk about how he dealt with being lonely. The little wounded part of him responded by telling a story:

> *Once there was a little boy who was lonely. He didn't like it. It hurt and was scary. He wanted the loneliness to go away.*

He put the loneliness in a box. It got out. He put it in a closet. It escaped. He mailed it to Antarctica. It came back. The little boy knew what he had to do. "I need to hide." And so he did. He hid in a dark place, far, far away. He was pretty sure he was safe from the loneliness. And he was. But he got lonely hiding. No one came looking for him. So he made a pretend little boy that he could hide behind. This pretend little boy was almost perfect. He didn't feel lonely or sad or anything but happy. The loneliness monster didn't hurt this pretend boy. No one could!

Of the many and varied emotions one can feel, love is undoubtedly the most healing, the most comforting, and the most nurturing. It is by far the most important emotion an adult survivor of childhood abuse can experience. There is no greater antidote to loneliness than love. And not surprisingly, this emotion is also one of the most difficult emotions to open up to and experience after having survived childhood trauma.

Love requires an openness—a vulnerability—that can be very difficult to achieve. For example, if I am hit repeatedly when my dad starts shouting, years later I will still flinch when a person raises his or her voice. This is an example of remaining on high alert. Being wary of when or where the next abusive act will happen, adult survivors are always tense, on edge. I often held my breath as an adult and tensed my muscles as if bracing for some kind of hidden impact that never came. I did it so much, I wasn't even aware of it until I started going to therapy. When it was pointed out to me, I was shocked to catch myself holding my breath repeatedly on any given day. Being so on-guard, how could anyone feel comfortable opening up?

Holding my breath and tensing up helped me to feel powerful. It reassured me that if I was going to be hurt, I was ready for it and therefore could do something to quash the threat. Survival became more important than love. It became more important than breathing. It became more important than living life.

Opening up to love can be seen as something dangerous, like letting knights lower the draw bridge as the enemy is advancing to attack the castle. Abuse can leave a person feeling used, dirty, or gross. When those acts are labeled love, the victim will come to associate love with feeling disgusting and gross inside. Love can be felt as oppressive and overwhelming, even suffocating. The mother who is in an enmeshed relationship with a son or daughter fosters the idea that love is heavy and draining. The child will feel overwhelmed with the oppressive and suffocating feelings they experience from their mother. There is no way a child can fill the empty space in a parent's heart. No child can fulfill the role of a spouse.

My Awakening to Love

I had a flashback in the evening hours of that summer day. It was about me and my abuser and the physical sensations I felt when she sexually abused me. The night of the flashback I had trouble sleeping. The next day I went crazy. I lost myself in one project after another. I pushed myself in a very obsessive manner to clean, to organize, and to rearrange the furniture. I started a big landscaping job and without much thought or planning invested nearly $1,000 in renovating part of the back yard for an eating area. By nightfall I was exhausted, yet when bedtime rolled around again, I still couldn't sleep.

I finally reached out to God. At first I was scattered and my words felt hollow. I stopped and tried to "get real" with Him. I told Him what was happening. I asked Him for help while I was sleeping, to help me in some way to heal and move beyond this one stuck moment in time. I prayed that maybe He could access a part of me that I couldn't get to in my awake state. I fell into a fitful slumber, never really getting into a deep, restful sleep. I remained on the cusp of consciousness, not quite asleep and not quite awake, for most of the night.

At one point, and I'm not sure if it was a dream or something else, I had the sense that my abuser was talking to me. She was telling me that this sensation—this overwhelmingly sensual, electric, heavy, take-my-breath-away kind of feeling was love. And then God was talking to me and told me it wasn't love—that what she was saying was a lie. He told me to reject this physical sensation, to say no to it. My abuser persisted in trying to persuade me. Heavenly Father kept encouraging me to say no and stand against it.

He reminded me of the many little and sometimes big experiences where I felt His presence. I was filled with a quiet, calm, solid sense of belonging. I felt as if I was bathed in warm white light, both inside of myself and outside. These sensations somehow made me feel more confident and stronger. In those moments there was no stuckness—no past experience that chained me down. In those moments I felt alive and hopeful. I had no worries about the past or the present. Heavenly Father asked me if I ever felt that way when my abuser sexually abused me. I said no.

Yet I was afraid. I was afraid to say no. I was afraid to stand against my abuser. I finally told God that this sensation I felt when I was abused was all I had that proved I was special. I believed these sexual acts were what gave me worth and value. It is why she picked me. These sexually abusive moments reaffirmed and validated my specialness.

Heavenly Father kept reassuring me that His love would never leave. Over and over He said that. And as He did, I felt all my muscles start to tighten. I practiced whispering the word no. And then I had this strange feeling that I was under water and had to rise up out of the water in order to say no. My muscles got tighter and tighter. I pushed against this heavy water-like sensation. Closer and closer I came to breaking the surface, with God constantly encouraging me. I could still hear my abuser's voice in the background, but it was getting fainter and fainter.

Suddenly, using all the force I could muster, I broke free and sat up in bed screaming "No!" as loud as I could. In that moment, as I yelled out that word, it was as if every cell, every muscle, joint, and ligament screamed it as well. Later I realized I wasn't just breaking out of the heavy, dark water I was buried in, but I was truly waking up from decades of being in a trance state—the fog, numbness, spacing out, disappearing, and dissociation.

All of me was saying no. The confused little boy was saying no. The terrified little boy was saying no. The little boy who wanted to believe the lie found in the seduction and abuse was saying no. And the adult me was saying no. There wasn't one part, one fragment, or one little piece of me that didn't—in that moment—hold back.

I was awake. I turned and sat on the edge of my bed, a little disoriented and not quite sure what to do. My wife was sitting in bed reading a book when this happened. "What was that?" she asked. "Are you okay? Did you have a nightmare?"

I couldn't find my voice, couldn't respond to her. My thoughts were jumbled. I lay back down in bed. She was quiet for a moment, watching me with deep concern. When I didn't say anything, she asked, "What's going on?"

And then I started to cry. I cried because I was sad—sad about the lonely world I grew up in. And then I was crying because I felt scared for being so emotionally "naked" and raw. All of these emotions swirled together. I tried to get a handle on them, but I couldn't. I tried to explain to my wife what I was experiencing, but the words came out in sobs and whispers.

Then I felt wave after wave of this peaceful, comforting, and soothing sensation from God. I cried as I felt that. I cried and cried.

Part of me wanted to stop and tell my wife what was going on, but I couldn't stop crying.

Finally I was calm enough to talk to her. As I did, I knew again that God was with me—that I could trust His love. All of me felt this truth. His love was as real and safe and perfect as my abuser's love was false and twisted and disgustingly selfish. My wife was very careful not to interrupt. She did not try to touch me or comfort me until I said it was okay.

This incident took three more days to "settle" inside of me. And when I woke up Sunday morning, I felt a happiness I had not experienced in a long time. It was not some kind of euphoric happiness a person might feel on Christmas morning, or on a first date with someone he or she had a huge crush on, or getting a bonus check in the mail. This wasn't a giddy, silly, or immature kind of happiness. This was a calm, solid, "I feel good" kind of happiness. And it didn't go away.

I spent the day in quiet reflection, in awe at God's love and how He really was there, deep in the trenches with me, fighting with me, and not ever leaving me. He answered my prayer. He heard me. He saw my distress. He never once abandoned me.

I had no idea what I was really praying for other than I knew I needed help that went beyond the mortal world that night. I almost want to say, as I look back on that prayer, that the idea of what to say didn't originate from me. Perhaps He told me what to say as I was praying. I do know that I had never prayed like that before or asked for something like that to happen to me before. It actually seems a bit odd, looking at what I asked for now. I asked for God to give me an experience in my sleep that would help heal me. I asked Him to reach in and work with the part of my brain I can't access while I am awake. And He did.

Love must be found. It is an essential part of accessing the Atonement. It becomes a way for Christ to heal us and make us whole. Therefore, it is no surprise that the adversary tries to keep us from finding love. But you can unwind your twisted beliefs about love. Have faith in God that He will keep you safe so you can open up to love. Allow the love from others inside—physically give it a place inside of you. And then express how it feels and what it does to you. Testify, sharing your experience with feeling loved. Then go out and express your honest emotions of love to someone else—your spouse, your children, your best friend. And love will be cleansed from the tar-like sludge of your abusive past, and become pure and full of light. It will become what it was supposed to be all along—uplifting, supportive, nurturing, ennobling, and strengthening.

Chapter 17

Fear

Not only does love require a physical and emotional openness, it also requires an individual to be "thawed out." When abuse strikes, one of the most common reactions in children is to freeze. There is little fighting back a child can do if an adult is hurting him or her. A child has very limited resources for help in fleeing from an abusive situation. Most children experience a sense of being trapped—being absolutely powerless—around people who are hurting them.

Over time, the child's heart remains "frozen." Walls are up, emotions suppressed, and we experience but a tiny fraction of our emotions. We become cardboard cutouts, full of superficial feelings. We can come across as aloof, cold, or very calm in a stressful situation. We're really just so detached that we couldn't react emotionally even if we wanted to. We may have a flat affect, meaning our faces reveal very little about how we are feeling. We may appear happy but feel hollow inside. And above all, there is an emptiness inside that never goes away.

When we feel a strong sensation, it can cause us to blank out or disappear. Sometimes we might describe ourselves as robotic, or dead inside. We may feel dizzy or feel as though we are slipping out of our body. These are all symptoms of freezing up as a result of childhood trauma.

Case Story

Jerry sat back on the couch, smoking a cigarette. I was sitting across from him in his house. He had the raspy voice of a chronic smoker, and a wrinkled face from working in the sun. He pushed his glasses up on his nose and moved his thick white hair out of his eyes. In an earlier session I had asked him questions about his past, but he had glossed over most parts. We were going back, trying to get a little more detail. With him being so blank and emotionally flat, something had to be missing.

"My mom and dad would go into town and I'd be left with the babysitter—a teenage girl from across the street. She'd always bring her friend along. I was probably five at the time, and pretty rambunctious. One time Jenny, the babysitter, took a rope and tied me up. Then she and her friend lifted me up and hung me on a meat hook that was hanging in the barn." Jerry took another long drag from his cigarette, not looking at me. He stared off into space.

"You mean they hung you up by the rope?" I asked.

"Hmm." He nodded. It seemed that was the end of the story.

"Well, how long did you stay there?"

"About four or five hours." His face remained passive. He put out his cigarette, looking as calm and serene as if he had just woken up from a long nap.

"So you hung there for four or five hours. On a meat hook. In the empty barn. Tied up. And you were about five years old."

"Uh-huh." Jerry acknowledged it as if it were nothing.

"Who found you?"

He seemed to think a moment before he said, "I'm not sure."

"Was it dark out?" I asked.

Jerry lit another cigarette. "Huh? Oh, yeah."

This is an example of dissociating. Jerry was telling about something terrible that happened to him, with the same kind of intensity a person might have in reading off a grocery list. He was as far removed from the experience as he could get. It turned out this was only the beginning of the torturous abuse he suffered. As more came spilling out, it became clear why he had disconnected from reality. He had needed to stop feeling. He needed to find a way to escape even when escape wasn't possible.

Jerry stayed in this numb state as the years went by. Now he was in his fifties, having lived a very hard life. He discovered he had to do more and more escaping from his past. The last thing he wanted to do was feel anything. So the smoking got worse. It was a great distraction for him. It calmed him down and helped take the edge off of his temper. Unfortunately, it was his blackouts that brought me to him. He would get so angry that he would black out and not be able to remember what happened.

How our bodies and brains choose to react to abuse becomes set—fixed. That means even as adults, we will often respond to highly emotional, stressful, or anxiety-provoking situations the same way we did when we were children. A child that responds to fear by freezing (literally rooted to one spot, unable to move, holding his or her breath) will experience that same reaction as an adult (unable to think, wide-eyed and unmoving, unable to find words to express himself or herself).

A child that reacts to fear by using the fight response—yelling, screaming, kicking, biting, and throwing things—will grow up confusing fear and anger. The fight response taps into the natural energy one feels when experiencing injustice. After repeatedly using this response to cope with fear, the fear may never be acknowledged. The individual will go straight to anger. As an adult, this person is short fused, has explosive anger, often destroys private property, gets into fights, yells a lot, and breaks into other's personal space to coerce and intimidate.

A child who uses flight (running away, hiding, trying to stay over at a friend's house for as long as possible, or getting lost in a fantasy world) as a way to cope with traumatic levels of fear will be twitchy and nervous. He or she always seems to be ready to burst into a run. This hyperactivity is sometimes misdiagnosed as a symptom of attention-deficit disorder rather than a result of trauma. An adult who uses this type of response to fear will use drugs, alcohol, and other addictions as a way to "flee" reality. They will run away from stress by quitting jobs, leaving relationships when things get tough, or becoming adrenaline junkies. Calm, peace, quiet, routines, and structure—all are seen as uncomfortable and undesirable. This person wants to keep running away—never facing the past or the present.

Fight, flight, or freeze—these are the three ways our bodies respond and react to traumatic fear. The emotion or sensation of fear is about experiencing an event that is life-threatening or overwhelmingly confusing and anxiety-provoking, all from a place of powerlessness and helplessness. This state of powerlessness increases and magnifies the fear.

While inborn, automatic response mechanisms assist us in surviving horrific events, when used repeatedly they can twist and distort the way we handle future fear. No one wants to feel this way again, so the focus of these reactive responses is to not feel fear. The abusive act is rarely the focus; rather, the focus is the powerlessness exhibited by the victim. These reactions promote the idea of trying to gain power over that which is causing the fear.

Power and Control

Jewel, a fourteen-year-old girl, had been sexually abused by one of her older brothers. I was working with her in a treatment facility for sexually reactive female adolescents. One day in group therapy, she talked about how her brother had taken away her power. "I felt powerless. I couldn't do anything. I needed to do something to get it back." She recounted how she'd flirt with older men and have sex with them. She felt wanted and desired and believed some of these men would do absolutely anything for her. She felt very powerful around them. Several of the other girls nodded. Referring to Jewel's comment about her brother taking away her power, I asked, "Can power be taken away?"

Sixteen-year-old Jewel, who had sexually abused her two younger cousins, raised her hand. "Sure. When I was raped I didn't feel I had any power. My uncle had all the power. You either have power over men, or they have power over you." Other girls agreed.

I handed four quarters to each of the girls. "Okay, let's go with your idea that power can be taken away. These quarters are your power. We're going to play a game. Every time you lose the round, you have to give a quarter to the person who won."

We played the game and after a few turns, Sheila, another resident, had amassed most of the quarters. "So Sheila, you took everybody's power away from them. And now you have a lot more power, right?"

She laughed and put her hands up in a victory stance. "Yeah!"

We played a couple more rounds, and suddenly Sheila went from having almost all the quarters to losing most of her money. "Oh, Sheila, what happened?"

She shrugged her shoulders.

"I lost."

I nodded. "And when you lost the game, you lost your power."

"No, I just lost some quarters," she said, obviously no longer wanting to associate the quarters with power. "You're the one who calls 'em power. Let's play some more. I'll get 'em all this time."

I asked her why, when she had most of the group's money, she had no problem referring to the quarters as power, but now when she was losing, she didn't want to. "Because I was winning. It was fun to take the quarters from everyone else."

And that was the point. "You're right. It is fun to win. But when you lose, it doesn't feel good, especially if we're playing with the definition that we lose our power each time we lose a quarter." I had the girls give back the quarters. I held the pile of change in my hands. "If this is my power, I will always be at the mercy of someone or something taking it away."

Andi broke in. "So you just have to be more careful. You've got to protect those quarters. Hide 'em or put 'em in a bank."

"And so I have to be always watching and do a lot to build up some kind of protection to keep my power safe."

Andi nodded her head yes. I jiggled the money in my hand, thinking for a moment. On the surface, what she was saying appeared to make sense. But that kind of thinking was what got the girls into trouble in the first place.

"Here's the problem," I said. "As long as we look outside of ourselves to measure and experience our sense of power, we will always be caught up playing the game. No matter how much you have one day, the next day something's going to happen and you'll lose it all. And if we're not playing the game, we're spending all our time trying to protect and guard our power."

I went on to discuss with the girls that just because we experience a moment of powerlessness while being abused does not mean the offender took away our power. Personal power is not something that can be given or taken away.

The concept of power can become skewed even if there is no overt abuse occurring in the individual's life. Powerlessness and not having control over one's life is a common variable in childhood. When one's primary caregiver is loving and nurturing and promotes a sense of security and safety, powerlessness is simply a developmental state that a child grows out of bit by bit.

However, if the primary caregiver has trouble allowing the child to take more and more power over his or her life, problems will occur. The child may become too dependent. As an adult, the individual may struggle with the concept of power and having a sense of control. These parts of the person's psyche will remain immature and underdeveloped. The flip side is also true. If the parent offers too much autonomy (encouraging control and a sense of personal power) before the child is ready, problems with limits, adhering to boundaries, and requiring the outside world to impose a sense of security and safety even in adulthood can result. Too much power before the child is ready can cause a deep sense of fear—even a sense of abandonment.

When a sense of powerlessness becomes integrated into a person's core concept of who he or she is, then love, esteem, and experiencing one's self-worth become conditional, based on whether or not the individual feels powerless or powerful.

For adult survivors of childhood abuse, powerlessness is almost always linked to believing that something bad is about to happen and that they are not safe. As soon as this idea occurs, they have a flight, fight, or freeze response. Most often, these moments of powerlessness occur when the individual is interacting with other people. In the moment, the adult survivor cannot see how extreme their reaction is.

The key to overcoming trauma-based fear is awareness and becoming present. As Stephen Wolinski states, "Feeling *current* restores one's sense of personal power and enhances one's ability to take responsibility for the ongoing moments of [present] experience(s)" (Wolinski, 1991). In other words, allowing ourselves to feel—to break out of the fight, flight, or freeze responses—allows us to become grounded in the here and now. Emotions are present-oriented. The more we can be in tune with our emotions, the more we can stay in the moment, and the less likely we are to overreact with a fear response. We want to react from today, not from twenty or thirty years ago when we were frightened children.

Learning to know what we are feeling helps us become more aware of ourselves. That awareness helps us to slowly but surely become comfortable in our bodies. If I can't escape the person who is hitting me, yelling at me, or touching me, I can at least escape from myself. Staying disconnected from our bodies as we grow up continues to be a hidden goal. Feeling, connecting to, and expressing our emotions bring us back into our bodies. It may be very frightening, but it is the only way we can truly heal.

In order to access the Atonement of Jesus Christ, we need to be emotionally aware and have the ability to stay in the present moment. We can't surrender something we don't own. We can't turn something over to God until we know what we have to turn over. There is a need to get to know the realness of our wounds in order to let them go. Let me be clear, however. There is no need to remain obsessed about the past. Remember, there is no healing by staying in the past. Healing can only happen in the present. The Atonement can only be accessed in the present moment of today.

Many years ago, I went to my older brother's funeral. I wanted to cry, but it wouldn't come. I felt a heaviness, but something stopped me from accessing that grief. Eight years later, as I started my journey of healing and recovery, I realized just how much I relied on my brother when I was little—just how much I needed him. Suddenly, the heaviness came loose and I started to cry. Finally, I was grieving. In order to access the grief bottled up inside me, I needed to connect to my brother's love and the other positive aspects of our relationship. I needed to connect to the past so I could feel the pain and grief. It is often the same for those carrying burdens of past trauma.

The principle of connecting to pain in order to heal is also part of true repentance. Alma reminds us of the need for godly sorrow—to feel physically uncomfortable about our actions, to experience emotional anguish. This is not because the Lord delights in our suffering, but because this type of pain is essential to receiving forgiveness. We need to be aware of what we have done, to understand the consequences, and to see our actions' ripple effects in other people's lives. Godly sorrow helps the repentant individual to understand why what he or she did was wrong, and why it is important to try as hard as possible to never return to that behavior again. There are only subtle differences between the process of repenting and seeking forgiveness, and the process of healing from our emotional and spiritual wounds of the past.

The prophet Lehi counseled his two elder sons: "O that ye would awake; awake from a deep sleep, yea, even from the sleep of hell, and shake off the awful chains by which ye are bound, which are the chains which bind the children of men, that they are carried away captive down to the eternal gulf of misery and woe" (2 Nephi 1:13). Most people assume Lehi is trying to get his sons to repent. Of course that is accurate. But consider how this verse relates to having experienced childhood trauma. Aren't we in a deep sleep—disconnected, detached, and in denial about our past? Doesn't this type of emotional, mental, and even spiritual sleep come from acts that originated from a hellish and sinful place? Aren't we bound by the chains of our pasts, still tied to the trauma of our childhood? Doesn't the past still impact our choices and cause us to handle life in maladaptive ways, thus filling our lives with misery and woe?

There is nothing quiet or subtle about breaking chains. We need to twist and torque and strain against them. We must be proactive to "act upon" the chains, as Lehi teaches us in the next chapter of 2 Nephi. Being acted upon and remaining passive will not yield the results of breaking free. We must bravely face the past. We must say, "No more! I will no longer let my life be dictated by the events of my past! I will stand up and confront the ghosts and demons of my past!" As we do, the Lord will be there to give us His strength, His courage, His insight, and His healing touch.

PART 4
CONCRETE TOOLS

Can a woman forget her sucking child, that she should not have compassion on the son of her womb? yea, they may forget, yet will I not forget thee. Behold, I have graven thee upon the palms of my hands; thy walls are continually before me. —Isaiah 49:15–16

Chapter 18
Session with Terri

Terri peeled an orange. She often brought one to her sessions. It gave her something to do with her hands, plus she really liked oranges.

"So how have things been going?" I asked.

"I'm feeling guilty."

"Oh? What about?"

Terri made a grimace and shook her head back and forth. "It's stupid," she finally said.

Not responding to her last statement, I waited as she ate the orange.

"I just . . . I just feel guilty about not taking care of the house like I should."

"Well, you are going through some pretty heavy stuff," I said.

"Yeah, but it's my fault."

"What is?"

"It's my fault the laundry isn't done. It's my fault we ate out the last three nights."

"But you're going through something really hard, Terri. Isn't it okay to have needs?"

She snorted and shook her head. "Oh, no, I'm not supposed to make more problems. I'm not supposed to make more work for other people," she said emphatically. "My mom taught me that."

I asked her what her mom did to make that clear.

"I haven't told you about this, but one of my earliest memories is when I was hungry and decided to make myself an egg. I got out the egg and the pan. I turned the stove on and tried to break the egg into the pan. Suddenly my mom started yelling and rushed into the kitchen. She grabbed me and yanked me away from the stove. She was really mad. She asked me what I was doing. I said I was hungry and wanted to eat an egg. I got sent to my room for playing with the stove."

"Why were you so hungry?"

"Mom had been sleeping in her bed all day. I was starving."

"How old were you?"

"Three."

"Did Mom do that a lot?" I asked.

"What?"

"Sleep a lot?"

"Yeah, she had just had a baby, but it died in the hospital."

"Oh. Sounds like she was depressed. Or grieving."

"Probably both," Terri replied.

"And here you were, three years old, having legitimate needs. You still needed to be taken care of, and your mother couldn't do it."

Terri didn't say anything, just nodded.

"Where was your father?" I asked

"He was going to school full-time. He'd leave in the morning and come home late."

"How long did your mom stay depressed?"

"Until she got pregnant again—when I was four and a half."

"So what did you do all that time?"

"Oh, I learned how to open the front door, and I would walk around the apartment complex saying hi to people."

"And your mother didn't know what you were doing?"

"No. Neighbors would give me food. They all said I was a very happy child. Very precocious. When my parents tell stories about our childhood, they laugh and think it was funny that I'd leave and go knock on doors and talk to people in the complex."

"So one of your earliest memories is trying to get your needs met and you got in trouble for it."

"Yeah, she was so mad at me for doing that," Terri said.

"Okay, but that was one experience."

"No, you don't understand. My mother would blame me for stressing her out, or for making her sad. I remember one day when my dad pulled me aside and said that my mother was crying in her bedroom and that it was my fault. He asked me what I was going to do about it."

"What did you do that made her cry?"

"I told her I wasn't going to babysit my younger brothers."

"How old were you?"

"Sixteen."

"How old were your brothers?"

"Seven and five."

"Why couldn't Mom take care of them?"

"She said she was too busy with her Church calling. I told her I was tired of always babysitting. I told her I spent so much time with my little brothers that they came into my bedroom at night when they had a nightmare instead of going into Mom and Dad's bedroom. I loved my brothers, but I wasn't the mother! I was done! I told her she needed to take more responsibility for the kids and that I was going to a school dance that night."

"So once again, when you had needs, you were made to feel bad. When you tried to stand up for yourself, you were given a guilt trip."

Terri nodded her head. "I've been on one long guilt trip my whole life."

"And that is why now, when you have real needs and you need help around the house, you feel guilty."

"Yeah."

"So let's try something. I'd like you to stand up and say in a forceful tone to your mother that you were hungry and she wasn't taking care of you. You were simply trying to feed yourself."

Terri looked embarrassed. "Do I have to stand up?"

"Yep."

She sighed and stood up. "Okay, what am I supposed to say?" I repeated it for her.

Terri rolled her eyes and started mumbling. I interrupted her. "No, be clear. Be bold. Stand up for yourself."

She sighed. "Do I have to?"

I nodded.

"Fine." She got a determined look on her face and said very clearly, "I was hungry. You weren't taking care of me. I was trying to make something to eat. You had been in bed all day. Then you got mad at me and sent me to my room. And I was still hungry!"

"Yes, that's right!" I encouraged Terri. "How does that feel?"

She looked at me, her eyes blazing, her hands in fists. Instead of answering my question, she continued to talk to her mom. "I was three years old! If you couldn't take care of me, you should have asked for help! I was left to scrounge for myself, basically going around and begging for food from the neighbors! And now you see that as a funny antidote! You took no responsibility for me then and you take no responsibility for your actions now! I am furious!"

I sat there, slowly nodding my head. "That's right," I said softly. "And you were never given permission to be angry about that."

"Of course not! Mom never wanted to hear anything real from me. She didn't want me to tell it how it really was. She couldn't take that. Remember, if she was upset, it was my fault." Terri pointed at herself, stabbing her finger into her own chest.

"So what do you want to say to Mom about that?"

"It wasn't fair! It wasn't right! How could I, a little girl, be responsible for your happiness? That was such a mean thing to do to me—such a heavy burden for me to carry!" Terri was shaking slightly, decades of anger shimmering off her. Hot tears of frustration rolled down her face.

"Do you want to keep carrying that burden?" I whispered.

She shook her head no.

"Then give it back to her," I suggested.

"Here, Mom, you take it all back—all your stress and anxiety that I had to take care of. It was yours—it *is* yours—and I don't want it." Terri pantomimed taking a heavy box off her shoulders and throwing it away. "I won't carry your guilt anymore!" She threw away more imaginary boxes. "I won't be responsible for your happiness anymore!" More boxes went flying through the air.

Terri suddenly broke down and started sobbing. She sat down on the couch and put her head in her hands. For a few minutes, we sat there as she cried. She eventually stopped and reached for a tissue. She blew her nose and wiped her eyes.

"How do you feel?" I asked.

"Shaky, but lighter."

"You let go of a lot of stored emotion."

"Yeah. It felt so real, too—like I was really unloading heavy stuff." She shook her head and gave me an awestruck look. "This stuff we do must look crazy to someone watching, but every time, no matter how crazy I think your exercises are, somewhere there is a click inside of me and it becomes real and I really get into it."

"You connected to your anger and pain and hurt and sadness and then did something physical while you were connected. It was real. How you feel right now is proof enough."

Terri blew her nose again, then sat back and sighed. "I am bushed. I feel like I just did a huge workout at the gym."

"Because you did do a huge workout," I said.

She nodded and stared at nothing for a few moments, her eyes unfocused. Then she turned to me and said with a clear voice, "It is okay for me to have needs."

"Yes, Terri. It is."

"And I don't have to feel guilty about having needs."

"No, you don't."

"Now I need a nap," she said.

I smiled. "Yes, you do."

Chapter 19
Overcoming the Natural Man

Abuse promotes a host of behaviors and beliefs that end up making it difficult to access the Atonement. As listed in chapter 3, these thoughts, attitudes, and actions limit agency and drive us farther from Heavenly Father. When King Benjamin declared that "The natural man is an enemy to God" (Mosiah 3:19), he was, from a therapeutic point of view, stating a basic truth. When we act from a broken, hurting place, our behavior reflects that place. When we sin, we are not in a righteous, whole, healthy state of mind. Just as peace creates peaceful actions, so too does anxiety produce anxious behaviors. Darkness creates dark choices and consequences.

In *Overcoming Addiction: A Twelve Step Companion Guide* (2011), as well as *Healing the Codependent Heart* (2013), I talk about the natural man, and how addiction and codependent behaviors thrive from this carnal, fallen state. We also end up in this state after we have been abused. For protection, we come to rely on ourselves and our own defenses. Trust diminishes. Stubbornness, pride, arrogance, and a refusal to look at our own actions become the norm. We become willful, controlling, and closed off to love. Everything goes through the filter of survival. People in a state of survival are of necessity selfish and unwilling to try new things.

Of course, the natural man can also look like the despondent, full-of-despair person. There is no hope and there is no faith. If tears are shed, they are not the kind that usher in soul-changing insight. They are tears of the beaten and broken who are trapped and stuck, seeing no way out. They are not tears that lead to godly sorrow. They are tears from the hopeless and helpless.

When we are in this natural state, it is pretty difficult to find Christ and healing. The adversary tells us to hold onto our outdated and distorted beliefs. He tells us the walls around our hearts will keep us safe. He whispers that we shouldn't hope because it will simply make us vulnerable and open to getting hurt again. He tells us to keep being workaholics, or alcoholics, or short tempered, or two faced, or codependent, or a sex addict—because all these behaviors keep us from feeling pain, facing our pasts, and healing.

In the short term, these actions work. We don't feel afraid. We don't feel pain. We can feed our egos and feel strong and invincible. In the long term, these maladaptive coping skills, rather than the abuse itself, actually become the thing that destroys us.

Therefore, it is essential for us to "yield to the enticing of the Holy Spirit," and "put off the natural man" (Mosiah 3:19) while we seek the healing powers of the Atonement. We can't find our Savior in sin, in dysfunction, or in the shadows. Amulek explains that Christ cannot save us in our sinful state:

> *And Zeezrom said again: Shall he save his people in their sins? And Amulek answered and said unto him: I say unto you he shall not, for it is impossible for him to deny his word.*
>
> *Now Zeezrom said unto the people: See that ye remember these things; for he said there is but one God; yet he saith that the Son of God shall come, but he shall not save his people—as though he had authority to command God.*
>
> *Now Amulek saith again unto him: Behold thou hast lied, for thou sayest that I spake as though I had authority to command God because I said he shall not save his people in their sins.*

> *And I say unto you again that he cannot save them in their sins; for I cannot deny his word, and he hath said that no unclean thing can inherit the kingdom of heaven; therefore, how can ye be saved, except ye inherit the kingdom of heaven? Therefore, ye cannot be saved in your sins.* (Alma 11:34–37)

Functional health cannot be found, created, or achieved while we live in a reactive, fragmented state of survival. Just as we must repent and stop doing our sinful behavior so Christ can save us, we must also try to handle our traumatic pasts differently so He can heal us.

"But I can't," you say. "I don't know how. I'm too scared. My patterns are too entrenched. I'm too full of anxiety when I try to handle life differently. You're asking me to get better before I can even heal." These are all statements I have heard, and some of them I have echoed myself. But just as repentance is necessary before baptism and receiving the gift of the Holy Ghost, we must open ourselves up to feel the Holy Ghost, follow His promptings, and recognize His inspiration before we can achieve healing.

This is not an impossible task. Remember, our brains are created to find health, healing, and the Atonement. Dr. Richard Davidson reminds us that "Based upon everything we know about the brain in neuroscience, change is not only possible, but is actually the rule rather than the exception. It's really just a question of which influences we're going to choose for our brain." (Davidson, 2013).

What we focus on changes our brain. When we focus on survival, our brain adapts accordingly. When we focus on not feeling emotions, our brain changes to accommodate us. When we focus on people-pleasing, enabling, or perfectionism, our brains rewire to support us.

It is also true that when we focus on spiritual matters, the brain helps us by searching for more spiritual connections. Why else do we hear over and over the need for daily scripture study and prayer? The more we put spiritual material into our souls, the more the whole organism changes to support that material. Let us not forget the power of grace, gratitude, and the admonition to hold fast as we try to refocus our attention on healing and living.

As hopeful as this information may be, it is almost always an uphill battle to change our focus. The pain and terror and confusion we felt when we were abused had to be intense enough to trigger automatic coping responses. If the abuse continued, the trauma changed our brain. That is what we are working against. "An experience repeated, the thousands of neurons that fired together and create the neural network of the initial response tend to fire again, strengthening that network and preparing the brain to respond in the same way when it next encounters a similar situation. . . . Neurons that fire together, wire together" (ibid, 10). This is referred to as conditioning. These neural pathways and patterns are stored in our implicit or unconscious memory. It is the foundation of what we call a "knee-jerk reaction."

Sounds hopeless, doesn't it? Ah, but the very same ability to create negative or trauma-based knee-jerk reactions can also create a knee-jerk reaction that causes us to do something healthy and proactive. We simply need to recondition our hearts and brains.

Remember, "no matter what the external trigger, it's our internal response, based on our neural wiring, that's important . . . Often we can't change the external stressor, but we can do something about our internal conditioned response to that stressor" (Graham, 2013, 12–13). This is hard to believe and have faith in. Trauma tells the victim that the threat is external—that it is out there. Therefore, we must remain ever vigilant of what's happening out there, or stay "asleep" (detach, disconnect, dissociate, deny) so we don't have to face the frightening aspect of being terrorized again.

Telling a victim of abuse that he or she can't do anything to change the external trigger—the external threat—is akin to people telling Christopher Columbus the world was flat and that his ships would sail right off the edge. It was the prevailing theory, and people thought he was crazy. Yet this notion is absolutely true. The earth is round, and it's our response to a trigger that needs to change, that can change—not the trigger itself.

I cannot change the external environment. Even as an adult, I have limited ability to neutralize an external threat. But I do have power to change how I will respond to that threat or trigger. Our brains were created to be adaptable. We can change our internal conditioned responses whenever we feel scared, anxious, powerless, helpless, or lonely. "Although the initial wiring in our brains is based on early experiences, we know that later experiences, especially healthy relational ones, can undo or overwrite that early learning to help us to cope differently and more resiliently" (Graham, 2013, 5).

How to Change Our Knee-Jerk Reactions

Being mindful and being empathetic are among the most powerful agents of brain change known to science. Both strengthen the functioning of the prefrontal cortex to rewire old patterns. This means that when we see a situation clearly (mindfulness or awareness) and accept compassionately what we are seeing (self-empathy), we can rewire old patterns without harming ourselves. God never talks about us hating ourselves if we sin or make a mistake. He never supports the use of self-pity or self-hatred as necessary requirements for change.

In most of the scriptures where Jesus Christ tells us He wants to heal us (see Doctrine and Covenants 112:13; Matthew 13:15; 3 Nephi 18:32; John 12:40), He pairs that desire with the need to become converted. In 3 Nephi 9:13–14, the Lord declares: "Will ye not now return unto me, and repent of your sins, and be converted, that I may heal you? Yea, verily I say unto you, if ye will come unto me ye shall have eternal life. Behold, mine arm of mercy is extended towards you, and whosoever will come, him will I receive; and blessed are those who come unto me."

According to the Bible Dictionary, conversion begins with a desire to follow and accept God's will. This change in attitude appears to be an essential and necessary requirement to access the Atonement and be healed. King Benjamin says we need to become submissive like a little child. Why is that such hard work? Because we've been children before, and terrible things happened to us when we were submissive to other adults.

So, we become willing to open ourselves to the enticing of the Holy Spirit. We open ourselves to truth, to experience awareness, and to be able to connect the dots and make sense out of our present maladaptive reactions to the daily struggles of life. We breathe, not from a shallow, ragged, fear-based place, but from our bellies. Our breathing will be full, opening us physically and emotionally and spiritually. We will follow the Spirit in becoming submissive—trusting God—willing to be humble and meek and patient. "For the natural man is an enemy to God, and has been from the fall of Adam, and will be, forever and ever, unless he yields to the enticings of the Holy Spirit, and putteth off the natural man and becometh a saint through the atonement of Christ the Lord, and becometh as a child, submissive, meek, humble, patient, full of love, willing to submit to all things which the Lord seeth fit to inflict upon him, even as a child doth submit to his father" (Mosiah 3:19).

In the end, we move from reacting to our pasts in a natural-man state, to becoming a saint through the Atonement of Christ. From this place, we have new tools to handle life. Our pasts are in our past. Our pain is healed. Our fear is taken away. Triggers may remain, but our reactions to them will change. And we are healed physically, emotionally, mentally, socially, and spiritually.

CHAPTER 20

GRACE

It is not uncommon for my clients to make comments about everything being too much—too much fear, too much pain, too much chaos and confusion. When they make such a comment, I agree with them. Sometimes they look at me strange, as if I was supposed to refute their statements. But what they are saying is true. Overcoming childhood abuse is a bigger task than anyone can handle alone.

Then I point out that in some ways, even though we are now adults and have resources at our disposal that we didn't have as children, we are still powerless over the past. When overwhelming trauma triggers the brain to compartmentalize, or dissociate from the unfolding event, reconnecting to the event years later can still cause the same reaction. Jumping back into the trauma is often retraumatizing. There is no healing inside of the emotionally infected wound of the past.

If the past needs to be reviewed, it is key to go there as an adult, instead of slipping back into a child state. Going there with a counselor is also critical. A therapist becomes the anchor to the present, with knowledge and ability to keep the client tethered to the present while sharing the truth of the client's past. And going there with God is key.

Why is that? Moroni explains that overcoming the stumbling blocks of this fallen world can be achieved by turning to God:

"And my grace is sufficient for all men that humble themselves before me; for if they humble themselves before me, and have faith in me, then will I make weak things become strong unto them" (Ether 12:27). Turning weakness into strength is what grace does. That is why having God with us as we travel the battle-torn paths of our past is essential—we need His grace.

Grace helps us to connect to the Atonement. It helps remove the aftereffects of abuse, both emotionally and physically. It infuses strength beyond our own, enlightens our minds beyond our own comprehension, and soothes the painful muscle memory of past abuse. Grace gives us hope when we feel hopeless. It pushes us out of bed so we don't miss our counseling session. It helps us rewire our brain, breaking apart old patterns that are outdated, twisted and distorted, and maladaptive. Grace gives us the courage to feel emotions, to get back inside our bodies and feel alive again.

Pray for grace. Ask for it, search for it, fast for it. And as Elder Richard G. Scott counseled: "Don't worry about your clumsily expressed feelings. Just talk to your compassionate, understanding Father. You are His precious child whom He loves perfectly and wants to help. As you pray, recognize that Father in Heaven is near and He is listening" (Scott, 2007).

A few days ago, I had a young man in my office who told me with an air of hopelessness that prayer didn't work for him. I asked him what he prayed for. He prayed for good things, but rarely was he specific. Rarely did he prepare himself before he prayed. And rarely did he wait and meditate a few moments after he prayed.

Be specific in your prayers. Prepare yourself before you pray. Think about what you want to say. Do some calming breathing techniques, like breathing in through your nose and out through your mouth, or breathing from your stomach instead of just your chest. Try to visualize Heavenly Father sitting with you. Now you are ready to begin praying.

As you pray, do so with real intent. This means to be honest, sincere, and willing to go and do whatever the Lord counsels you to do. Talking about your emotions is a good way to get to that honest place. Explaining what you are thinking and what is happening at that moment can also help.

What should we pray for? We should pray for grace. We should pray for spiritual power beyond our own to help us overcome the debilitating effects of abuse. If we have been blinded by the past, we should pray for the spiritual gift of awareness and insight. If we have been hardened by the past, we should pray for a spiritually softened heart. If all we see is despair and darkness, we should pray for the spiritual gift of Christlike hope. President George Q. Cannon taught:

> *If any of us are imperfect, it is our duty to pray for the gift that will make us perfect. Have I imperfections? I am full of them. What is my duty? To pray to God to give me the gifts that will correct these imperfections. If I am an angry man, it is my duty to pray for charity, which suffereth long and is kind. Am I an envious man? It is my duty to seek for charity, which envieth not. So with all the gifts of the Gospel. They are intended for this purpose. No man ought to say, "Oh, I cannot help this; it is my nature." He is not justified in it, for the reason that God has promised to give strength to correct these things, and to give gifts that will eradicate them.* (Cannon, 1894)

At the end of your prayer, try to do the same things you did to prepare yourself before the prayer. Then move forward. Sometimes answers come immediately. Sometimes they come later in the day as you continue to meditate on what you were praying for, or they come while you are driving to the store. Sometimes answers come from other people. They may come from your counselor, your bishop, your spouse, or even your child. President James E. Faust stated: "Each of us has problems that we cannot solve and weaknesses that we cannot conquer without reaching out through prayer to a higher source of strength. That source is the God of heaven to whom we pray in the name of Jesus Christ" (Faust, 2002). Hold onto those words when answers don't seem to come right away.

With every tiny step you take that leads you to Christ, you will be blessed with grace. In fact, even before you have the energy to move, grace will be there. LDS scholar Brad Wilcox explains that "Grace is not a booster engine that kicks in once our fuel supply is exhausted. Rather, it is our constant energy source. It is not the light at the end of the tunnel, but the light that moves us through the tunnel. Grace is not achieved somewhere down the road. It is received right here and right now" (Wilcox, 2012).

So many of us deal with and manage our past trauma in maladaptive ways. Trying to alter our reality and escape the pain and fear within us, we turn to food, gambling, sex, drugs, alcohol, and even prescription drug abuse. When we are riddled with sin, we often want to withdraw from the Lord instead of turning to Him for help. And then, even when we want to turn to Christ, our attempts are filled with false starts. Elder Bruce C. Hafen offers us some comfort as we search for grace even as we struggle to remain obedient to the commandments:

> *The interaction between our efforts and God's grace is represented by the covenants of the Atonement, described in the sacrament prayer. Our part of that covenant is not that we may never make a mistake; it is, rather, that we are* willing *to take upon ourselves his name, willing to always remember him, and* willing *to keep his commandments . . . . On this condition, he will always*

> *be with us, to heal, to compensate, to strengthen us by the gifts of his Spirit—for those gifts are 'given for the benefit of those who love me and keep all my commandments,* and those that seeketh so to do' (D&C 46:9; emphasis added). *The Lord offers the gifts of the Spirit not only to those who* do *but also to those who, willing but struggling,* seek to do *his will.* (Hafen, 2008)

Case Story

"Your heart is like a sponge," my therapist said. "It soaks up feelings, experiences, all sorts of stuff. And just because your heart soaked up some icky stuff doesn't make you icky or bad. Your heart was just doing what hearts do."

She had me look at my heart. There was thick, black gunk. We tried to collect it, but it was so attached to the muscle tissue that it was ripping my heart as I tried to remove it. She tried another tactic. She asked if we should clean little Doug's heart. I said yes. I imagined shimmering, translucent blue water cascading from my head and down into my body. It swirled around my heart, and the black gunk eventually disappeared. Then I realized there was another deposit in my stomach. It was larger and harder—like a rock. The cleansing water did nothing to it. Then the therapist had me imagine light coming from heaven, entering my head, and slowly moving through my body, cleansing and sanctifying it. The light got to my stomach, but all it did was crack the hard, black sludge into little bits.

My counselor asked me as the adult to say something to the little part of me. After I said a quick prayer, the following words just flowed out of my mouth. "I accept you. I accept your pain. I accept your terror. I accept your confusion. I accept all parts of you." The Spirit flooded over me, and with tears running down my cheeks, I felt light. Then the color changed to a brightness—a white light that seemed to come from within and expand. The sensation was akin to feeling the Spirit, but it was also burning away the chunks of filthiness. The sensation filled me and then it was done.

I had tears, but they were tears of joy. I felt a magnificent peace come over me. The thought came to me: "I know what you don't. I took you where you needed to go to continue your healing and to find a deeper peace." Heavenly Father did for me what I could have never done on my own.

This story from my own journey shows the power and reality of grace. Grace is essential. It is necessary and it is real. I have seen the impact and effects of grace not only in my life but in the lives of countless brothers and sisters trying to overcome their childhood abuse. Believe. Reach out. Try. He who trod the wine press alone will be there with you.

CHAPTER 21
GRATITUDE

Another crucial element in accessing the healing power of the Atonement is gratitude. As with most of the keys we have discussed, gratitude can be a difficult attribute to foster when working to overcome childhood abuse. Often, we are acknowledging pain, fear, guilt, and shame. We are trying to manage waves of anger. We are hit with heavy sadness, mourning the losses that accompany abuse. There is nothing light and airy when we are in the midst of facing our traumatic pasts. In this state of mind, it can be tough to find things to be grateful for. Yet, as Elder Quentin L. Cook of the Quorum of the Twelve Apostles declared, "We should be grateful for all the tender mercies that come into our lives. We are unaware of hosts of blessings that we receive from day to day. It is extremely important that we have a spirit of gratitude in our hearts" (Cook, 2011).

Lance was a client who came to see me because of his anger issues. This brother in the Church had almost no self-esteem and was very thin-skinned. His reactions were often over the top. He almost always interpreted others' statements the wrong way. For him, everything was an attack on his level of competence. He lost jobs over it. He lost friends because of it. He was on the verge of losing his wife. He came into my office one day and sat down, already in a bad mood.

"Okay, you wanna know my secret?" he asked me.

"Sure."

"I can't read."

"That must be hard for you. How do you manage at work?"

"I watch what the other guys are doing and then repeat what they do." He shrugged his shoulders. "I'm good with my hands, and I pick things up fast."

"I don't doubt it," I said.

Lance fiddled with his boot laces, clearly nervous about telling me his secret.

"What happened when you were a child?" I asked.

He licked his lips and swallowed. "I wasn't good at reading."

"Well, did the school help you?"

"They tried, but I would just clam up."

"Did your mom help you?"

Lance snorted. "My mom? Oh yeah, she helped me," he said, his words dripping with sarcasm.

"What do you mean?"

"I'd come home with books to read. I tried to hide them from her, but she'd find them and make me sit down at the kitchen table." Lance bunched his hands into fists and pounded the chair he was sitting in. "I hated it so much! I'd be sitting there wincing, waiting for the slap to come."

"The slap? Did your mom slap you?"

"Yeah. If I couldn't get a word right, she'd slap me. Mother would struggle through a few minutes with me and then lose control. She'd chew me out—calling me names, swearing at me, telling me I was worthless and stupid." Lance's face was red, and it looked like he was holding his breath.

"Breathe," I said softly. The trapped air came out of his mouth with a *whoosh*. "That's right, keep breathing as you feel these emotions."

"I wanted to tell her she was wrong—that I wasn't worthless. I was trying!" Lance shook his head back and forth, almost like he was trying to shake the memories out of his head. "And you know what they found out later on? Years later? That I was dyslexic! It wasn't that I was stupid—it was that I was dyslexic!"

His voice rose higher, his eyes grew wider, and he spit out each word as if they were laced with vomit. "I! Was! Dyslexic!"

"Breathe," I encouraged again. He tried, but his breaths came out ragged and shallow. He started to talk again, but I motioned for him to be quiet. "Just sit for a moment and breathe," I directed. Twice more he started to ramp up, and twice more I guided him back to his breathing. After a few minutes, Lance's face wasn't red anymore. He slumped back into the chair, looking exhausted.

"She would slap me and accuse me of faking. She called me lazy."

"How did that make you feel," I asked quietly.

Tears welled up in his eyes. "I was so scared. I was so lonely. I was so confused. The words never made sense. The letters were always jumbled up. It didn't matter if I tried to sound them out, everything was gibberish."

"Why are you crying?"

"Because I'm angry."

"Anything else?"

"Hurt."

I nodded. "You were hurting. And you still are."

Acknowledging that broke something in Lance and he started to sob. He cried and cried. It was the beginning of his healing.

To help him with his dark view of the world, I had him make gratitude lists. He always fought me on it. It seemed almost painful for him to think that way. He couldn't write, so I'd have him tell me ten things he was grateful for. Sometimes they were silly answers. Sometimes they were more heartfelt. Then I started having him do a list with his wife, before he left for work and before he went to bed.

Over time there was a subtle shift. Lance smiled more. He was able to handle compliments better. He wasn't as angry or as critical, and he didn't have such strong reactions. Many things that helped him, but I believe gratitude was one of the first steps in helping him to unlock his wounded heart and become more open to Christ's love.

Why gratitude? Because biologically, we function better when we experience and express gratitude. We were created to be creatures of gratitude. Heavenly Father knew the horrible events we would have to suffer. Not only did He create automatic survival programs in our brain to protect our psyche from abuse, but He also made it so our brains and hearts could heal from that abuse by way of experiencing gratitude.

Dr. Alex Korb explains the biology of gratitude.

> *Researchers at the National Institute of Health examined blood flow in various brain regions while subjects summoned up feelings of gratitude (Zahn et al, 2009). They found that subjects who showed more gratitude overall had higher levels of activity in the hypothalamus. This is important because the hypothalamus controls a huge array of essential bodily functions, including eating, drinking and sleeping. It also has a huge influence on your metabolism and stress levels. From this evidence on brain activity it starts to become clear how improvements in gratitude could have such wide-ranging effects from increased exercise, and improved sleep to decreased depression and fewer aches and pains.* (Korb, 2012)

Dr. Korb goes on to explain how gratitude also triggers the brain to release dopamine. "Dopamine feels good to get, which is why it's generally considered the 'reward' neurotransmitter. But dopamine is also important in initiating action. That means increases in dopamine make you more likely to do the thing you just did. It's the brain saying, 'Oh, do that again'" (ibid).

From this, we can see that gratitude begets gratitude. Optimism flourishes. Compassion and empathy flow from being grateful. The old messages and destructive patterns of the past slowly melt away as new patterns emerge, urged on by the good feelings from dopamine. Dr. Korb calls this a virtuous cycle. He states,

> *Your brain only has so much power to focus its attention. It cannot easily focus on both positive and negative stimuli. It is like a small child: easily distracted. Oh your tummy hurts? Here's a lollipop . . . On top of that your brain loves to fall for the confirmation bias—that is, it looks for things that prove what it already believes to be true. And the dopamine reinforces that as well. So once you start seeing things to be grateful for, your brain starts looking for more things to be grateful for. That's how the virtuous cycle gets created.* (ibid)

If I believe I will be hurt again, the brain will look for future threats. If I believe I am worthless and unlovable, the brain will look for evidence to support that belief. If I believe I was made to be a sexual object, my brain will look for repeated confirmation of that belief. And this focus will influence my behaviors.

Similarly, the more we look for gratitude, the more the brain will focus on it. And gratitude begets humility. Gratitude begets joy. Gratitude begets hope. Gratitude begets charity. Gratitude opens the door for us to feel and see the effects of grace in our lives. We begin to see more and more of God's hands in our lives. Whereas we once may have doubted He even thought about us or cared about us, now with gratitude we start to see His tender mercies on a daily basis.

We are literally wired to directly access the Atonement. Our brains were made to connect to the effects of Christ's ultimate sacrifice. Our brains are made in such a way that as we try to live basic gospel doctrines, actual physical changes occur. The physical impact of past trauma in the brain is reversed. Healing happens. The principle of gratitude is just one example of how this occurs.

It's easy to start. Make gratitude lists, like Lance did. Pray for gratitude. Look for at least one piece of evidence that shows you that Heavenly Father loves you and is aware of you each day. When I was working through my past, sometimes I would walk outside and spend five minutes studying, feeling, and smelling the rose bushes outside my house. I began to experience a profound sense of awe for these flowers. This awe turned to wonder, which turned to a heart full of gratitude for these roses. God created these roses so that their fragrance and beauty could comfort my wounded soul. According to Byron R. Christensen, former president of the Halifax Nova Scotia Temple, "It's the little things that will bring us to the cure—that will bring us to Christ" (Christensen, 2013).

This may be a hard thing to read, but at some point there will be gratitude in your heart for the journey you have walked. At some point, you will look back and see how much the Lord has changed you, molded you, loved you, and cleansed you from the evil effects of your childhood abuse. At some point, you will echo the words of Shane, a client I worked with. One day, he said simply, "I'm grateful for the blessing of this trial." When I asked him why, he explained that in working to overcome the trial, he found Jesus. "For that reason alone, it was worth it. I wouldn't have made the sacrifices to find Christ if I didn't have to. I don't think anyone would. But life was too crazy, too chaotic, too full of despair. I couldn't keep living like that. So eventually I became willing to do whatever it took to find peace."

"And did you?"

With tears in his eyes, he nodded. "I finally felt His love. It was the most real spiritual experience I've had. I know my Father in Heaven loves me. I know my Savior loves me. And I have been changed because of that. I will always be grateful for walking the path."

Shane put his missionary papers in soon after we ended therapy. He served a two-year Church mission and spent his time testifying to others of the reality of God's love for us. After Shane came home, he told me with a big smile, "I am so glad I went through hell to find God." I laughed and we embraced, fellow travelers searching for Christ.

While a member of the Quorum of the Twelve Apostles, James E. Faust gave comforting words to those who have gone through great trials to find God: "Out of the refiner's fire can come a glorious deliverance. It can be a noble and lasting rebirth. The price to become acquainted with God will have been paid. There can come a sacred peace. There will be a reawakening of dormant, inner resources. A comfortable cloak of righteousness will be drawn around us to protect us and to keep us warm spiritually. Self-pity will vanish as our blessings are counted" (Faust, 1979).

CHAPTER 22

FORGIVENESS

Of the numerous things a person can do to heal from past trauma, forgiveness remains one of the most powerful. Many times clients will reference Doctrine and Covenants 64:10—"I, the Lord, will forgive whom I will forgive, but of you it is required to forgive all men"—and then say they have no idea how to forgive their abusers. Often the offenders are family members, and the effects of their behaviors on my clients have been enormous. Most abused individuals realize that forgiving the abuser is essential to obtaining healing from the Lord, but because this is such an overwhelming thing to do, they believe they will be lost forever.

One such client had many people to forgive. Her bishop and stake president kept encouraging her to forgive these individuals. She knew it was the right thing to do, but she had no idea how to actually go about it. "The Primary answers aren't enough," she said. This wasn't forgiving someone because they stole her parking space at the mall. This wasn't forgiving her child for throwing blocks and breaking her favorite lamp. No, this was something much deeper, much heavier, and much more profound.

From our discussion, we drew up a detailed step-by-step process by which she could genuinely and authentically forgive people who caused her so much emotional and spiritual damage. Notice that these steps are not simple and cannot be completed in a few minutes. There is a need to experience a real shift and do a lot of healing work before the final step can be achieved. Some steps may take days, weeks, or months. Yet by doing them, we can truly and fully forgive the people who hurt us so profoundly. And we will experience the promised blessing of feeling free from our past.

1. Acknowledge the wound. See it, understand it. Know its story.
2. Acknowledge the feelings of the wound. Allow it to have a place in your life—don't run from it, shun it, ignore it, or bury it.
3. Share my feelings with God. Admit to Him that the pain, hurt, and injustice are too big for me. Admit that if I try to stay in control of the wound, trying to manage something this big could destroy me.
4. Pray and ask for the pain to be removed from my heart. I need to have an attitude of acceptance about the past and becoming willing to give up all the defenses I created to protect the wound and stop the pain.
5. Ask and seek the Lord for comfort and protection. I need Him physically by my side when I am around people who hurt me or people that remind me of my past abusers. I give up my defensive mechanisms and let the Lord become my Defender and Protector.
6. With humility, ask the Lord to show me my sins, inadequacies, and character defects. Repent of them. At some point, I need to acknowledge that my survival coping mechanisms had a negative impact on others. I need to move from focusing on what happened to me, to concentrating on my own behaviors.
7. Contemplate Mosiah 2–5. This is King Benjamin's great discourse. I need to look for insight from his discourse

that will help with my healing and forgiveness for my own sins and other's sins.

8. Feel God's love for the people that hurt me. It may not be possible for me to generate love towards them. I need to become open to feel God's love for them. I come to love them with godly love, meaning charity.
9. Officially forgive the people who hurt me. Most of the time that is a personal experience between me and God.
10. Endure to the end. Maintain charity by staying close to the Savior. See the love God has for each of us.

As I am writing this book, this dear sister is still working through these steps. She does not see this list as daunting or impossible to achieve. Rather, she is grateful she now has a map to help her find what she has been so desperately searching for. I routinely remind her that she needs to use the other parts of accessing the Atonement to help her—grace, gratitude, and overcoming the natural man.

During our journey toward healing, there will be moments where we must make a choice: either stop and fixate on the unfairness and injustice of what has happened to us, or move forward to forgiveness. Both choices have emotional and physical consequences. "Brainwaves slow to a grind and serotonin supplies diminish under excessive weights of a grudge . . . If you repeatedly find yourself drowning in a sense of injustice or bitter disappointment—you may create a pattern of bitterness" (Weber, 2011). There is no healing in seeking justice. Only as we search for mercy will the Atonement cleanse us and heal us from the past.

Remember that our brains were engineered to connect to the Atonement. Forgiving is a part of the Atonement. As we choose to forgive others, forgiveness "literally alters the brain's wiring—away from distortions brought about by the past, and beyond fears that limit the future. It leads from misery of a broken promise, to wellness that builds new neuron pathways into physical, emotional and spiritual well-being. Forgiving brains fuel unconditional love. How so? Speak of another's genuine value, rather than replay disappointment's darts—and sorrow fades from the brain's amygdala, like clouds float off on a sunny day" (Weber, 2011).

Forgiveness is not to be taken casually or lightly. It requires sincere effort. And it must not be rushed. It is not the first, second, or even third thing to do in overcoming our traumatic pasts. Many times, Church leaders instruct members to forgive spouses, parents, siblings, or even other members of the congregation. This is a noteworthy and accurate piece of counsel. Sometimes, however, the member doesn't know how to get from where they are, to where their bishop wants them to be. Confused, the member leaves with less hope than he or she had before entering the bishop's office. Just because the counsel goes right to the end of the story doesn't mean it is bad advice.

At some point, all victims will be asked to see their offenders in a different light. Many who have relished in the idea that their offenders will endure the justice of God and burn in hell will need to change their thinking. We don't wait to forgive until our offenders own their behaviors, or take responsibility for what they did, or even come out and apologize. We don't wait for justice to come before we forgive. We forgive as soon as we are ready to take that step. We forgive even if our offenders are still being unsafe and acting in dysfunctional patterns. There is never, ever a justifiable reason to place expectations or conditions on our decision to forgive. Elder Renlund reminds us:

> *As God encourages us to keep on trying, He expects us to also allow others the space to do the same, at their own pace. The Atonement will come into our lives in even greater measure. We*

> *will then recognize that regardless of perceived differences, all of us are in need of the same infinite Atonement . . . My invitation to all of us is to evaluate our lives, repent, and keep on trying. If we don't try, we're just latter-day sinners; if we don't persevere, we're latter-day quitters; and if we don't allow others to try, we're just latter-day hypocrites. As we try, persevere, and help others to do the same, we are true Latter-day Saints. As we change, we will find that God indeed cares a lot more about who we are and about who we are becoming than about who we once were.* (Renlund, 2015)

Seek for grace and gratitude as you work toward forgiveness. It will come. With it, the peaceful realization that you are free from the past will fill your entire being. You will become a living witness to the power and majesty of the Savior's great sacrifice.

PART 5
THE BOOK OF MORMON

Behold, the Lord hath shown unto me great and marvelous things concerning that which must shortly come, at that day when these things shall come forth among you. Behold, I speak unto you as if ye were present, and yet ye are not. But behold, Jesus Christ hath shown you unto me, and I know your doing. —Mormon 8:34–35

Chapter 23

Session with Terri

As Terri walked into my office, I immediately knew she was doing better. There was something different about her.

"How are you?" I asked.

"I've been working out—going to a gym—and I have a trainer!" she said excitedly.

"That is awesome." I had been encouraging her to become more physically active to help with the depression and grief she was feeling from her childhood.

"But boy, oh boy, I'm really sore from my workout."

"Oh really?"

Terri ran her hand down the back of her leg. "My hamstrings are really sore. My trainer says they are wound really tight."

"Do you think there is a connection between your abuse and your muscle soreness?"

"Of course." Terri seemed a little put off by my question. "Don't you remember when we talked about how my physical pain often triggers me, making me more nervous and anxious?"

I nodded my head. "You have definitely held a lot of stored emotion in various parts of your body."

"It's the same kind of pain I felt back in high school when I'd stretch before basketball. It filled me with incredible fear and anxiety then, just like it does now." Terri closed her eyes and hugged a pillow on the couch. It looked like she was about to fall asleep—about to dissociate. "Terri, open your eyes."

"No."

"Yes, open your eyes."

"I don't want to," she whined.

"Why not?"

"Because then you'll tell me to feel my feelings, and I don't want to feel them."

"What's wrong with feeling your feelings?"

"They make you go back." By now Terri did have her eyes open. I decided to try a different tactic.

"Have you ever seen a movie?" I asked.

"Uh-huh."

"And if it was a sad movie, did you feel sad?"

"Uh-huh."

"How long do you think that sadness stayed with you?"

"About five minutes."

"And then what?"

"Then I went back to feeling normal."

I nodded my head. "So that is what memories are like. They are movies about you—about something that happened to you. Sometimes you will feel feelings about what you are seeing. But just like your sad movie, these emotions will also pass."

Terri shook her head. "No they don't."

"Our job is to acknowledge, to feel the emotions, and they will pass. When we try to deny them or ignore them, they end up trying to get our attention. If we feel them and get lost in them, we will feel stuck and overwhelmed. Feelings are not meant to stay. They are not meant to be pushed down and kept behind a locked door. They are meant to be experienced, and then they leave."

"No way."

I tried a different tactic. "Terri, why do you think your hamstrings are so tight?"

"Because I'm scared when I feel those muscles."

"How come?"

"Because I'm afraid someone will hurt my bum."

"Like when the clown man raped you."

Terri's eyes flashed with anger. "Don't say that! Shut up!"

"Is that what you mean?" I ignored her flash of anger, knowing it was her usual way of trying to change the subject.

"Yes, but don't say that!"

"Can you show me what the exercise stretch is that causes you to feel so anxious?"

Terri rolled her eyes and started to whine and complain. Then she paused, her face becoming determined. "No, we're not going to fight against this," she said to herself. She got up and started moving her leg, doing her stretch.

"Now, as you do your stretch, tell yourself that you accept the memory your muscle is sharing with you."

She squirmed, and it was clear there was a struggle going on inside of her. Finally she repeated the statement. I had her repeat it over and over while she continued to stretch. "Keep doing your stretch. Remind yourself this is 2015. You are an adult. There is nobody behind you that is going to hurt you."

Terri repeated the words. Her little voice started to protest, but I interrupted. "It's 2015 and my trainer is safe." And her trainer was safe. It was a female friend from church whom she had known for several years.

Terri repeated the statement.

I went back to the first statement I had her repeat. "I accept what my muscle memory is telling me."

This shut Terri down. She sat back down on the couch in a huff. "I will not accept what happened to me."

"Accepting is not the same as liking it or saying it was okay."

Begrudgingly she said, "I accept what happened to me even though I hate it."

"Okay. That's okay."

Terri gave a short laugh. "Well, that's the only way I'm going to be able to get myself to say it."

"You have a lot of emotion about what happened," I said, trying to reflect what she was experiencing at that moment.

"I feel a lot of hate. A lot of anger." She picked up a pillow off the couch and thumped it on the ground. "I. Didn't. Like. It," she said, smacking the pillow on the ground with each word.

"You accept what happened as a part of your life story, and you are angry it happened." She repeated what I said and hit the floor with the pillow.

"And I want to be free of the past—free of being constantly dragged back to these scary moments."

"Yes!" she said loudly, whacking the floor again. "I want my life back! I am tired of being hijacked by my past!"

"For that to happen you will one day forgive your abusers."

This made Terri pause. "What? No way."

I cupped my hands as if I was holding some water in them. "Sometimes forgiveness can be as simple as filling my hands up with anger and vengeance and giving it to the Lord. It doesn't mean I have to face my offenders. It doesn't mean I tell myself it wasn't that big of a deal. It does not mean I am okay with what they did. I don't have to do some big religious ceremony. I can simply find that anger, find that desire for vengeance, and turn it over to God."

Terri thought about what I had just said. She started talking to herself, as if she were a parent talking to a child. "No, we're not going to freak out. We can listen to this. We want to be free. One day we will do whatever we need to in order to be free. No, that is not what Doug is saying. Forgiveness does not mean we are okay with what happened to us. It means we are letting go."

She got quiet and let go of the pillow. She had a thoughtful expression on her face. I waited and watched her. She took a couple of deep breaths and then looked at me. Her eyes were clear, and her facial muscles looked relaxed.

"I feel better," she stated. "I feel lighter."

I nodded, smiling. "You were able to connect memory, emotion, and your physical body in what you did today. That often helps us to release stored or stuffed emotions. You look more serene."

She nodded. "I feel it. And boy, what a workout!"

"You may need a nap later on today," I suggested.

Terri smiled. "Oh, I already had that scheduled even before the session started." We laughed together.

CHAPTER 24

AN ESSENTIAL TOOL FOR HEALING

For adult survivors of childhood abuse, the Book of Mormon is one of the greatest resources available to aid in healing. Elder Jeffrey R. Holland made this powerful statement in general conference:

> *I testify that one cannot come to full faith in this latter-day work—and thereby find the fullest measure of peace and comfort in these, our times—until he or she embraces the divinity of the Book of Mormon and the Lord Jesus Christ, of whom it testifies. . . . God always provides safety for the soul, and with the Book of Mormon, He has again done that in our time. Remember this declaration by Jesus Himself: "Whoso treasureth up my word, shall not be deceived"—and in the last days neither your heart nor your faith will fail you."* (Holland, 2009)

The Book of Mormon was written for us, in our day, to help us overcome the trails and tribulations of our times. Childhood abuse is one of the most prevalent scourges of our day. In our healing, we need the inspiration of the Book of Mormon. We need the blessings promised to those who study it. We need its peace and hope and its power to disperse the darkness.

I had read the Book of Mormon many times, but it took the words of inspired Apostles to help me finally see how it provides the way to overcome the effects of abuse. The Book of Mormon became my guide for healing and recovery. I could find metaphors, analogies, and direct statements that spoke to this journey of repentance and redemption. It was like reading the book for the first time. I was seeing what I had never seen before.

As with all sin described in the Book of Mormon, there is always an accompanying prescription for overcoming it. The prophet Alma states that "the chains of hell which encircled them about . . . were loosed. And their souls did expand, and they did sing redeeming love. And I say unto you that they are saved" (Alma 5:9). Here we assume the prophet was referring to sinners, but his words could also be said to define the state of abused individuals and what happens as they overcome the effects of that trauma.

Then Alma asked this great question, which I asked myself as I was reading. "How are they saved? What is the cause of their being loosed from the bands of death, yea, and also the chains of hell?" (Alma 5:10). He explains that these people who were in this awful condition:

- Were taught the words of the prophet Abinadi about the Atonement
- Humbled themselves
- Put their trust in the true and living God
- Received a mighty change in their hearts—became spiritually born of God
- Held out faithful to the end—continued to repent.

The book of Mosiah became one the greatest parts in the Book of Mormon for me as I worked on overcoming my past. In this book are found the words of Abinadi, the great discourse of King Benjamin, and the story of Alma the Younger and his miraculous conversion. All have such direct application to people on the road to recovery and healing.

One of the stories I have read and reread was of the bondage and eventual freeing of the people of Alma the Elder from Amulon and the Lamanites. Abridging the plates, Mormon explained that Alma and his people were "in bondage, and none could deliver them except it were the Lord their God" (Mosiah 24:21).

The people had been in bondage for years, building houses, growing crops, and tending to their herds. They were oppressed and beaten down. The Lord performed a great miracle to deliver them, putting all the Lamanites into a deep sleep that lasted all night and the next day. They were in such a state that even when Alma's people moved their herds, their families, and their grain, the guards did not wake up. Then the Lord stopped the Lamanites from pursuing Alma's people in the wilderness. Their escape and freedom was assured.

How many times had I told myself I was stuck, chained to my past? No matter what new calling I received, which new ward or city we went to, the past followed me. I simply could not move forward in my journey of healing. When I read Mosiah 24, I knew I was in bondage and no one—not the bishop, my wife, my therapist, my sponsor, books written by experts, or myself could free me from this bondage. It was bigger than me—than all of us.

Then the phrase "none could deliver them except the Lord their God," echoed over and over in my head. There was hope! I could find peace. I could be freed from the chains of the past. It was God who could and would do it. That is the power of the Book of Mormon.

The next three chapters will focus on 2 Nephi 2. I believe the powerful concepts in its verses can give us hope and strength as we seek to heal from an abusive past.

Chapter 25
A Father's Counsel: 2 Nephi 2

The prophet Nephi declared, "For I did liken all scripture unto us, that it might be for our profit and learning" (1 Nephi 19:23). Following that pattern, I will liken to us the precepts found in 2 Nephi 2. In this chapter, Lehi and his family have just crossed the ocean to the promised land. Lehi knows he will soon die. Reflecting on his family and their lives, he counsels his son Jacob.

2 Nephi 2:1

And now, Jacob, I speak unto you: Thou art my first-born in the days of my tribulation in the wilderness. And behold, in thy childhood thou hast suffered afflictions and much sorrow, because of the rudeness of thy brethren.

Here Lehi describes to his son Jacob what many have experienced—struggles and trials, and for many of us, trauma that happened during our childhood. One of the saddest points the great patriarch makes is that his son's "afflictions" occurred because of family members.

One of the great regrets of Lehi's life, it seems, is that within his own family—the family of a prophet—violence and terror raised their ugly heads. Laman, Lemuel, and some of the sons and daughters of Ishmael repeatedly threatened, physically harmed, and otherwise abused Nephi and those that followed him, and more than once brought the entire family to the edge of death.

Jacob was born into this kind of setting—one that included fear, intimidation, a keen sense of powerlessness, and brutal violence. Remember that his father, Lehi, was old when Jacob was born, and became more and more frail as the journey to the promised land continued. Laman and Lemuel were strong and had most of the family on their side. Even if Jacob wanted to stand up to these merciless bullies, he would have been outnumbered.

Within days of Lehi's death, Laman and Lemuel attempted to murder Nephi and Jacob and the rest of the family that followed after them (see 2 Nephi 5). This act underscores just how dangerous and volatile the situation was. As Elder Joseph B. Wirthlin declared, "If Satan can weaken or destroy the loving relationships among members of families, he can cause more misery and more unhappiness for more people than he could in any other way" (Wirthlin, 1993).

Many of us were born into situations where our own parents struggled under their own "days of tribulation." Sometimes our parents could do little more than keep their own heads above the rising flood of turbulence and chaos in their lives. Sometimes they were the ones who ended up hurting us—afflicting us and causing us "much sorrow." Sometimes it is a brother or a sister, an uncle or a grandparent. Sometimes it is the school bully, or the babysitter. Countless people can tell stories that match and sometimes exceed that of Jacob.

It is interesting that Lehi started out his conversation with his son Jacob in this way, addressing the boy's travails and burdens. But the great patriarch immediately offered spiritual reassurance, saying that all would be for Jacob's benefit. Perhaps Jacob wondered why he was born into a family where his brothers wanted to murder him.

As we begin our journey of healing and recovery, many of us come to see the reality of what was and what is. When this awareness comes to us, we often ask the "why" questions. Thanks to modern revelation, we know that when we came to earth, we were not born into our families by random chance. Elder Robert C. Oaks of the Quorum of the Seventy said:

> *Elder Russell M. Nelson of the Quorum of the Twelve Apostles came to conduct an area training session. During that session Elder Nelson made a statement that resonated in my heart then and continues to do so today. He said, "Understand who you are in God's plan." This powerful concept should be a major objective of our lives here in mortality . . . We are each individuals with singular talents, strengths, opportunities, and challenges. We believe we were foreordained to come to earth at a particular time into particular circumstances and that our particular set of gifts, attitudes, and talents—if properly developed and employed—will enable us to fulfill a foreordained purpose. (Oaks, 2008)*

A woman once asked her stake president, Dr. Carlfred Broderick, a world-renowned family therapist and member of the Church, the same question. This was his reply:

> *Where is the justice? How can God pretend to be just and send some little girls into homes where they are loved and . . . made to feel like somebody and others into homes where they are beat and molested and abused and neglected? What did I do in the pre-earth life to deserve such a family? I felt inspired at that time to tell her that she had volunteered in the preexistence to be a savior on Mount Zion, to come to a family drowning in sickness and sin and to be the means of purifying that lineage. Before her in that line were generations of ugly, destructive family relationships.*

Downstream from her purifying influence every generation would be blessed with light and love. The role of a savior, I said, is to suffer innocently for the sins of others that still others may not suffer. There can be no higher calling. She knew by the Spirit that what I suggested was true. That perspective gave her the strength to get on with her life . . . I suspect that many of us, more than most would ever guess, have made such pre-mortal choices and accepted such divinely demanding missions. (Broderick, 2008)

There is much hope in Dr. Broderick's words. Many of the families we come from have a history of dysfunction. To see ourselves as breaking not only the chains of our own past, but the chains of past and future generations, is encouraging and ennobling. Jacob was able to do this. He broke the chains of his own torturous past and taught his son Enos to love the Lamanites, who included Enos's uncles and cousins and who wanted to destroy the Nephites from off the face of the earth.

2 Nephi 2:2

Nevertheless, Jacob, my first-born in the wilderness, thou knowest the greatness of God; and he shall consecrate thine afflictions for thy gain.

Let's take this amazing promise apart. What does it mean when Lehi says that the Lord will consecrate Jacob's traumatic past? To consecrate means:

- To make or declare to be sacred
- To set apart, dedicate
- To sanctify something by setting it apart
- To solemnly dedicate or devote something or someone to a sacred purpose

Another way to phrase this promise is that the Lord will set apart, sanctify, and dedicate Jacob's "affliction" for his gain. This impending stumbling block will be turned into a wealth of opportunity and growth. The potentially destructive force that could lay waste to his heart and soul will be transformed into rich and fertile spiritual ground. His wounds will be turned from weakness, a handicap, to greater emotional and spiritual strength.

This verse brings a sense of relief to the weary and offers hope to the fallen. To know that as we come to see and feel and understand the "greatness of God" in our own lives, the trauma of the past will no longer trip us up in our quest for health and wholeness. Instead, Heavenly Father will turn our afflictions into an invitation to come unto Christ and be partakers of the Atonement. That means that my suffering, your suffering, does not have to be an end to itself. It does not have to be a dead end that cuts off all forms of escape from a life filled with distress, disappointments and despair.

We can rejoice as our hearts are healed and as we receive strength beyond our own ability through the grace of Christ. We can shout for joy as we are given insight and knowledge as to how to break the patterns of the past. We can turn to God with full trust, knowing He will take care of us and be our Protector. Truly our weaknesses will be made into strengths.

Lehi goes on to instruct Jacob about the Atonement—why we need this great sacrifice and how to access its blessings. The rest of the chapter will build on the hope and comfort you have received from the first few verses.

2 Nephi 2:5

And men are instructed sufficiently that they know good from evil. And the law is given unto men. And by the law no flesh is justified; or, by the law men are cut off. Yea, by the temporal law they were cut off; and also, by the spiritual law they perish from that which is good, and become miserable forever.

The law of justice requires perfect behavior—always choosing the right. There is no option to deal with bad choices, poor decisions, or mistakes. Within the law of justice, healing and recovery do not exist. There is no chance to try again and again. From justice's point of view, any sin will eternally separate us from God.

2 Nephi 2:6–7

Wherefore, redemption cometh in and through the Holy Messiah; for he is full of grace and truth.

Behold, he offereth himself a sacrifice for sin, to answer the ends of the law, unto all those who have a broken heart and a contrite spirit; and unto none else can the ends of the law be answered.

We can never be saved by trying to live according to the law of justice (see Romans 3:23–24; Galations 2:16, Mosiah 13:28). So how can we be saved? How can we be reunited with Heavenly Father? Verse 6 states that redemption comes because of Jesus Christ. Verse 7 explains how—Christ's sacrifice answered the requirements of the law of justice, allowing us the chance to be saved. Joseph Walker explained:

The gift of repentance is possible because of the atonement of Jesus Christ. Everyone who has ever sinned—and that includes all of us—needs to remember this. Since "there cannot any unclean thing enter into the kingdom of God" (1 Nephi 15:34), and since we have all become spiritually unclean because of sin (see 1 John 1:8), none of us would be worthy of exaltation without benefit of the Savior's intercession. Christ said, "For behold, I, God, have suffered these things for all, that they might not suffer if they would repent; But if they would not repent they must suffer even as I" (D&C 19:16–17). (Walker, 1992)

There is only one caveat. The ability to access this gift only comes if we have a broken heart and a contrite spirit. In other words, the Atonement—a chance to repent, a chance to experience healing and recovery, a chance to be saved even in our mortal state—only works for those who offer a broken heart and a contrite spirit to the Savior.

One brother, who used food as a way to manage his childhood abuse, was given the understanding of how his food addiction affected him spiritually. He explained how he saw a broken heart as someone who is open and vulnerable, feels emotions, and has a softened heart instead of a hard heart. He saw how his eating disorder kept him from feeling emotions—it kept him numb and sedated, kept his heart closed. He explained how a contrite spirit is someone who is humble, is teachable, and has a repentant attitude. This man's eating disorder kept him from experiencing humility.

He said, "I am still going after my way to solve problems and find protection and comfort. I turn to my 'god'—my food—to meet my needs. It keeps me in a prideful state. I am not submitting to Heavenly Father or His ways. I follow after Satan's counterfeit of peace and comfort."

This brother's compulsive overeating kept him from accessing the fullness of the Atonement, leaving him to his own devices, and to the law of justice. There can be no true healing or lasting peace for this dear brother, because as long he remains outside the boundaries of the Atonement, he is in the grasp of justice. And justice does not offer healing. Justice does not offer hope or mercy or grace. Justice cannot offer recovery or change. This man will remain stuck—in a state of perpetual relapses and binges—until he submits and offers his will to Heavenly Father.

2 Nephi 2:8

Wherefore, how great the importance to make these things known unto the inhabitants of the earth, that they may know that there is no flesh that can dwell in the presence of God, save it be through the merits, and mercy, and grace of the Holy Messiah, who layeth down his life according to the flesh, and taketh it again by the power of the Spirit, that he may bring to pass the resurrection of the dead, being the first that should rise.

Understand this one point—the Atonement of Jesus Christ is the only way we can access the benefits of healing and change. Healing and recovery exist only as we qualify for the blessings of the Atonement, which requires a broken heart and a contrite spirit. Without a penitent heart, the blessings of repentance, of healing and recovery, of a change of our very nature, can never happen.

2 Nephi 2:9

Wherefore, he is the firstfruits unto God, inasmuch as he shall make intercession for all the children of men; and they that believe in him shall be saved.

What does Lehi mean when he says Christ "shall make intercession for all the children of men?" To intercede means to plead or make a request in behalf of another, or to intervene for the purpose of producing an agreement—to mediate. Elder Yoshihiko Kikuchi of the First Quorum of the Seventy stated: "The prophet Abinadi explains that Jesus Christ's intercession means 'standing betwixt [the children of men] and justice; having broken the bands of death, taken upon himself their iniquity and their transgressions, having redeemed them, and satisfied the demands of justice' (Mosiah 15:9)" (Kikuchi, 2004).

I have led a life filled with constant stops and starts as I struggle to shake free of the chains of my abusive past. Without the Savior interceding on my behalf, I will remain in these chains and will never be able to become free. I will never be able to be reunited with my Heavenly Parents. I will be Satan's forever. He will own me and I will become like him—miserable and damned. The chains of my traumatic childhood, without this intercession, will reach out through the eternities, binding me and imprisoning me forever.

Christ steps in and says to our Eternal Father, "I vouch for this man (woman). I have paid the price required by the law of justice for this brother (sister)." Jesus then turns to us and says, "My dear brother (sister), you are now mine. As you make the sacrifice of a broken heart and a contrite spirit, and live within that spiritual state, you will be able to go where I go, live where I live, and enjoy the sweet reunion with your eternal Heavenly Parents as I have."

Lehi ends this verse by restating that there are bounds within which the Atonement works in terms of forgiveness and eternal life: "And they that believe in him shall be saved." Abinadi echoes this statement with even more clarity. He explains that Jesus Christ's Atonement was made for "His seed," or "heirs of the kingdom of God" (Mosiah 15:10–11). "For these are they whose sins he has borne; these are they for whom he has died, to redeem them from their transgressions" (Mosiah 15:12). And how do we become a part of that group? We offer up the sacrifice of a broken heart and a contrite spirit. In verse 28, Lehi encourages his children to do just that.

2 Nephi 2:28

And now, my sons, I would that ye should look to the great Mediator, and hearken unto his great commandments; and be faithful unto his words, and choose eternal life, according to the will of his Holy Spirit.

Lehi then introduces Jacob to the law of opposition. I can only imagine how this topic was received, with Jacob having experienced opposition in an extreme manner during his youth. Seeing it from a spiritual point of view probably gave him a deeper understanding, and perhaps an acceptance of what he had suffered.

Many times as I waded through my own afflictions and sorrows, I half jokingly thought maybe I had made a wrong choice in supporting Heavenly Father's plan of salvation. In the moment of stress and pain, Satan's plan appears a bit easier to swallow. How many times have you wondered, "Why all the abuse and turmoil? Why do I have to go through such difficulty? How come healing from the wounds of the past is so hard?" Understanding the law of opposition can help us answer these questions.

2 Nephi 2:11

For it must needs be that there is an opposition in all things. If not so, my first-born in the wilderness, righteousness could not be brought to pass, neither wickedness, neither holiness nor misery, neither good nor bad. Wherefore, all things must needs be a compound in one; wherefore, if it should be one body it must needs remain as dead, having no life neither death, nor corruption nor incorruption, happiness nor misery, neither sense nor insensibility.

2 Nephi 2:12

Wherefore, it must needs have been created for a thing of naught; wherefore there would have been no purpose in the end of its creation. Wherefore, this thing must needs destroy the wisdom of God and his eternal purposes, and also the power, and the mercy, and the justice of God.

Here we find one of the greatest lines in all of scripture—"For it must needs be that there is an opposition in all things." But what does it really mean? Since before the foundation of the world there have been opposing forces—good and bad, light and darkness, sickness and health, heat and cold. These forces exist independent of what we do.

Opposition gives us a setting where choice—agency—can exist. Agency was present in the premortal realm, as was opposition. Agency is present here on earth, as is opposition. Agency will be present in the spirit world after death, as will opposition. Simply put, without a state of opposition, there is no choice, for we would have nothing to choose from. The late Apostle John A. Widtsoe stated, "It is because of this eternal 'opposition' that man is able to choose, thus doing good or evil" (Widtsoe, 1943).

The survival techniques we use to manage the effects of our abuse eventually become a stumbling block to accessing the Atonement. We seek to create an artificial environment or reality where opposition is suspended. We attempt to wipe out anything that opposes happiness or euphoria. We desires to erase hurt, sadness, guilt, awareness, fear, anxiety, difficulty, struggles, and trials. But if we try to remove opposition, choice or agency will disappear as well. We cannot have one without the other. If I live my life trying to subvert the law of opposition, I also subvert my agency.

Elder D. Todd Christofferson of the Quorum of the Twelve Apostles explained: "Satan has not ceased his efforts 'to destroy the agency of man.' He promotes conduct and choices that limit our freedom to choose by replacing the influence of the Holy Spirit with his own domination (see D&C 29:40; 93:38–39). Yielding to his temptations leads to a narrower and narrower range of choices until none remains and to addictions that leave us powerless to resist" (Christofferson, 2009).

In every setting of our existence, there are stretching moments, experiences that push us out of our comfort zone. Dealing with opposing forces challenges us, tries us, and in the end, helps us grow. It may be intellectual, as in learning new mathematic equations. It may be emotional, as in experiencing an event that may feel overwhelming. It may be spiritual, where we have to reach out and use our faith in a way we never have before. It may be physical, where we go beyond what we previously thought was our limit, as in running a marathon or lifting weights.

Sometimes, especially during this fallen mortal existence, opposition can look like being born with a deformity, or struggling with a learning disorder. This type of opposition does not have to be the result of someone else's choices. There are healthy cells and healthy development as well as sickness and mutations.

Other forms of opposition are a direct result of someone else's choices. Evil begets evil. Wounded people wound people. In these circumstances, the consequences of one can be felt by another. I can be affected by someone else's sins. Sexual, physical, and emotional abuse create incredible obstacles for the victim. But as with other types of opposition, the person will have the choice as to how to deal with the experiences.

Chapter 26

A Father's Counsel Continues

Continuing to speak to his son Jacob, Lehi explains another universal law—that all of God's creations can either act or be acted upon. This law is tied directly to the law of opposition. Lehi tells Jacob that acting (in this sense, making a choice) can only occur when a person is "enticed" by one choice or the other. These choices are often opposites.

2 Nephi 2:13–16

And if ye shall say there is no law, ye shall also say there is no sin. If ye shall say there is no sin, ye shall also say there is no righteousness. And if there be no righteousness there be no happiness. And if there be no righteousness nor happiness there be no punishment nor misery. And if these things are not there is no God. And if there is no God we are not, neither the earth; for there could have been no creation of things, neither to act nor to be acted upon; wherefore, all things must have vanished away.

And now, my sons, I speak unto you these things for your profit and learning; for there is a God, and he hath created all things, both the heavens and the earth, and all things that in them are, both things to act and things to be acted upon.

And to bring about his eternal purposes in the end of man, after he had created our first parents, and the beasts of the field

> *and the fowls of the air, and in fine, all things which are created, it must needs be that there was an opposition; even the forbidden fruit in opposition to the tree of life; the one being sweet and the other bitter.*
>
> *Wherefore, the Lord God gave unto man that he should act for himself. Wherefore, man could not act for himself save it should be that he was enticed by the one or the other.*

Maybe we are in the grocery store, feeling hungry, and a thought flits through our mind to grab a candy bar and eat it quickly before anyone notices. For an adult survivor of abuse, whenever we feel or experience something that reminds the brain or body of the abuse, we have a "knee-jerk reaction." We react, often employing a host of coping skills that we may not even be consciously aware of. For most of us, the reaction is a foregone conclusion. Often these reactions become overwhelming to the point of "needing to" or "having to" act on them. Why? Because in that reactive state, we have slipped back or regressed to a younger state and see only three possibilities—fight, flight, or freeze. In that moment, we lose our sense of agency.

Whenever we try to escape opposition, we simultaneously limit our agency—or even lose it entirely. Trying to sidestep opposition often leads us from acting to being acted upon; from a fighting, survivor state to a victim state; from being assertive to becoming passive.

Here is another way to look at this. If I try to escape opposition by allowing myself to be acted upon instead of acting, I will:

- Continue to run and hide from my past, refusing to see it or deal with it
- Keep my addiction a secret, if I have one
- Refuse to accept the past

- Refuse to soften my heart
- Remain a victim
- Not stand up to those who hurt me
- Accept put-downs, intimidation, and coercion

On the other hand, if I accept that opposition exists, I am willing to accept my past as it was, not I as wanted or hoped it would be. I will be able to acknowledge to pain of my past and not fight against it. This level of acceptance will actually help me become more connected to my agency. With more agency, I am able to act. I will:

- Face my abusive past
- Get professional help as needed
- If necessary, go to a support group
- Speak the truth about my past and present
- Forgive my abusers
- Become a survivor
- Live a life based on principles that promote a functional and healthy state
- Be assertive
- Say no to abusive situations and people

2 Nephi 2:17–18

And I, Lehi, according to the things which I have read, must needs suppose that an angel of God, according to that which is written, had fallen from heaven; wherefore, he became a devil, having sought that which was evil before God.

And because he had fallen from heaven, and had become miserable forever, he sought also the misery of all mankind. Wherefore, he said unto Eve, yea, even that old serpent, who is the devil, who is the father of all lies, wherefore he said: Partake of the forbidden fruit, and ye shall not die, but ye shall be as God, knowing good and evil.

Lucifer's desire was to destroy agency as well as opposition. This would mean abolishing these universal laws. There would be no sin, no suffering, no opposing forces, and no choice. His selling point? No one would be lost—all of his fellow brothers and sisters would return to Heavenly Father's presence.

On the surface, this doesn't sound that bad, does it? No one gets left behind. Mortal life would be a cake walk. We wouldn't have to worry or struggle. We would get our bodies and make it back to God's presence. How could Heavenly Father even want to promote a plan where He would risk losing His children? Elder Bruce C. Hafen of the First Quorum of the Seventy explains:

The process of becoming Christlike is a matter of acquiring skills more than a matter of learning facts and figures. And there is something about the nature of developing those divine skills that makes it impossible even for God to teach us those things unless we participate in the process. We shouldn't expect it to be otherwise—what piano teacher could teach people to play if they were unwilling to practice? What coach could improve the capacity of an athlete without supervising the athlete's own trials and errors?

The idea that salvation is a process of skill development may help us to understand why there is a veil. We need not be impatient that things must be the way they are—we should, rather, be grateful. These circumstances show us how faith and repentance and knowing God are processes and principles of action, understood not by defining them but by experiencing them. God is a great teacher, and he knows the patterns and the principles that we must follow in the active conduct of our lives

> *in order to develop divine capacities. He can teach it to us—he has that power—but only if we will give ourselves to the process.* (Hafen, 1977)

So many times therapists tell their clients to "trust the process," or "stop fighting and give yourself to the process." For those of us wishing to heal from our traumatic pasts, the process is that of applying the Atonement in our lives.

What did Lucifer want in exchange for saving us? He wanted all of the honor and glory. He wanted to take his place on God's throne and become the most powerful being in the universe. Lucifer desired for every soul to bow down and worship him:

> *Behold, here am I, send me, I will be thy son, and I will redeem all mankind, that one soul shall not be lost, and surely I will do it; wherefore give me thine honor.*
>
> *Wherefore, because that Satan rebelled against me, and sought to destroy the agency of man, which I, the Lord God, had given him, and also, that I should give unto him mine own power; by the power of mine Only Begotten, I caused that he should be cast down;*
>
> *And he became Satan, yea, even the devil, the father of all lies, to deceive and to blind men, and to lead them captive at his will, even as many as would not hearken unto my voice.* (Moses 4:1, 3–4)

Because Lucifer's plan was thwarted and he was cast out, never to obtain a physical body, he fights unceasingly against the Father and the Savior Jesus Christ—and against all of us who chose to follow the Father's plan. Lucifer's goal is to create misery and despair in our lives. As we read in the Book of Mormon, "Satan did stir them up to do iniquity continually; yea, he did go about spreading rumors and contentions upon all the face of the land, that he might harden the hearts of the people against that which was good and against that which should come" (Helaman 16:22).

What more perfect way to continue his rebellion against the Father than with the tool of abuse. Childhood abuse destroys agency. Reacting from a place of raw emotion causes us to seek ways to thwart opposition. The Apostle Peter's description of the adversary creates a vivid picture and reminds me of how it feels to be in the clutches of my abusers—being hunted and devoured: "Be sober, be vigilant; because your adversary the devil, as a roaring lion, walketh about, seeking whom he may devour" (1 Peter 5:8).

Make no mistake—Satan, the father of all lies, is also the father of all abuse. This should come as no surprise, as the weapon of lies and the weapon of abuse always go together. Abuse is a fertile breeding ground for lies—not just the lies our abuser tells us, but those we tell ourselves in order to survive. These lies masquerade as truths, yet whatever may have been true at the moment we were abused, that truth is not necessarily reflected in today's reality. Whenever we try to use our childhood truths to explain our current, adult situation, we call it a distorted truth. As Lehi reminds Jacob, Satan tempted Eve in the Garden of Eden by telling her half truths, successfully enticing her to follow him instead of obeying God's law. President James E. Faust said that "These subtle entreaties make Satan the great imitator, the master deceiver, the arch counterfeiter, and the great forger" (Faust, 2007).

As we listen and act on the adversary's lies, becoming more and more entrenched in our reactive, maladaptive behaviors, there is a spiritual consequence. "We all have an inner braking system that will stop us before we follow Satan too far down the wrong road. It is the still, small voice within us," President Faust explained. "But if we allow ourselves to succumb to Satan's tempting, the braking system begins to leak brake fluid and our stopping mechanism becomes weak and ineffective" (ibid). This is why we struggle to connect to, have faith in, and use the Atonement to help us heal from the past. The more we use willful, mortal-based ways to deal with our abuse, the more immune we become to the whisperings and gentle nudges of the Holy Ghost.

2 Nephi 2:21–25

And the days of the children of men were prolonged, according to the will of God, that they might repent while in the flesh; wherefore, their state became a state of probation, and their time was lengthened, according to the commandments which the Lord God gave unto the children of men. For he gave commandment that all men must repent; for he showed unto all men that they were lost, because of the transgression of their parents.

And now, behold, if Adam had not transgressed he would not have fallen, but he would have remained in the garden of Eden. And all things which were created must have remained in the same state in which they were after they were created; and they must have remained forever, and had no end.

And they would have had no children; wherefore they would have remained in a state of innocence, having no joy, for they knew no misery; doing no good, for they knew no sin.

But behold, all things have been done in the wisdom of him who knoweth all things.

Adam fell that men might be; and men are, that they might have joy.

Elder Melvin J. Ballard, a member of the Quorum of the Twelve Apostles from 1919 until he passed away in 1939, explained the necessity of repentance during morality:

It is my judgment that any man or woman can do more to conform to the laws of God in one year in this life than they could in ten years when they are dead. The spirit only can repent and change, and then the battle has to go forward with the flesh afterwards. It is much easier to overcome and serve the Lord when both flesh and spirit are combined as one. This is the time when men are more pliable and susceptible. We will find when we are dead every desire, every feeling will be greatly intensified. When clay is pliable it is much easier to change than when it gets hard and sets. (Ballard, 1922)

Because of the Fall of Adam and Eve, we had the opportunity to be born into mortality. Lehi goes even further, though. He says that our existence—our *raison d'etre,* our purpose for being—is to experience joy. How many times I have read "Men are that they might have joy" and thought that Lehi got it wrong, that my existence is not filled with joy—in fact, it is often quite the contrary. But I did not understand.

Before the Fall, there was no mortality, no death, no sin, no excitement, no boredom, no sadness, no joy. There was opposition, as Lehi taught (remember the two different trees in the Garden of Eden) and there was agency (God allowed them to "choose for themselves"). But until Adam and Eve made their own choices pertaining to God's laws, the first man and woman on earth lived in a "bubble" of sorts, protected from consequences and trials—and unable to progress.

Because of the Fall, I had the opportunity to be born, and so did you. And just as Adam was, we are left with a choice. What will we do? Whom will we follow and listen to? Because of the Fall, when we came to earth, we entered a state where there was no neutrality. We could feel a thousand different sensations. We could experience many different moods and emotions. We could, in this state, feel joy. Joy can exist when its opposing force, sadness, exists as well. Because of that opposition, we can learn and grow, which is the purpose of this mortal life.

It's okay to feel sad. It's okay to feel guilty. It's okay to feel angry and scared. Why? Thinking back to Lehi's words, we know that each emotion is linked to and exists because of its opposing emotion. Whereas the adversary wants me to focus only on the joy, the happiness, the ultimate high, Heavenly Father knows I cannot experience true and lasting joy or peace or serenity unless I am open to all emotions. Part of having a broken heart, after all, is a feeling heart—an openness and a willingness to experience the bitter as well as the sweet.

After all that Jacob had already endured in his young life, this message was a powerful one. Lehi was basically telling his son not to harden his heart and build up walls and defenses and withdraw from love and life because of what he experienced. In fact, Lehi was admonishing his son to do the opposite—to love even more, to be even more open to God and the Savior, to reach out more and succor those that suffer as he did.

This is an important part of the message of healing and recovery. We are all "recovering'" our lives from the emptiness and isolating effects of our abusive pasts. We are "rediscovering" our emotions. We are being "restored" and "reclaimed" by our loving Father in Heaven through His Only Begotten Son's great and eternal sacrifice.

CHAPTER 27

A FATHER'S FINAL PLEA

The prophet Lehi reminds his son Jacob that because of our agency—because we will all make bad choices and commit sins—we need to be redeemed from the Fall. That redemption comes through the infinite Atonement of the Messiah, the Lord Jesus Christ. But Lehi offers this caution, and I paraphrase: "My son, you will be able to act for yourself—make your own choices—but you cannot choose the consequence of those choices. You will not be acted upon, except when you break God's commandments. Then the consequences will come and will act upon you. Because you and I are mortal and imperfect, we sin and make mistakes, so please repent. Seek the Messiah so He can intercede on your behalf and you can gain eternal life."

2 Nephi 2:26–27

And the Messiah cometh in the fulness of time, that he may redeem the children of men from the fall. And because that they are redeemed from the fall they have become free forever, knowing good from evil; to act for themselves and not to be acted upon, save it be by the punishment of the law at the great and last day, according to the commandments which God hath given.

Wherefore, men are free according to the flesh; and all things are given them which are expedient unto man. And they are free to choose liberty and eternal life, through the great Mediator of all men, or to choose captivity and death, according to the captivity and power of the devil; for he seeketh that all men might be miserable like unto himself.

A client once asked me how he ever had the chance to be free and "choose liberty and eternal life," since he had suffered severe abuse at an early age, which put him on a course of self-destructive, addictive behaviors. As we talked, we reviewed this chapter and pointed out a phrase which resonated with my client. He said, "Oh, there is that little phrase—'through the great Mediator of all men.' As I come unto the Savior, He can offer me freedom. He can restore me to a state of liberty and agency." And so it is with all of us.

2 Nephi 2:28–29

And now, my sons, I would that ye should look to the great Mediator, and hearken unto his great commandments; and be faithful unto his words, and choose eternal life, according to the will of his Holy Spirit;

And not choose eternal death, according to the will of the flesh and the evil which is therein, which giveth the spirit of the devil power to captivate, to bring you down to hell, that he may reign over you in his own kingdom.

In verse 29, Lehi gives his son a key concerning Satan's power. He tells Jacob that the "will of the flesh" is what gives the adversary the power to trap us and chain us and reign over us. Satan knows that to capture the spirit, he must first chain the body. Is it any wonder that abuse alters our state through physical means? Every type of abuse changes our brain chemistry, alters our neural pathways, and slowly destroys our physical bodies. Those changes support the continued use of survival-based mechanisms well after the need for those skills are needed. That is why they become maladaptive and dysfunctional. The Prophet Brigham Young declared, "Now I want to tell you that he [the devil] does not hold any power over man, only so far as the body overcomes the spirit that is in man, through yielding to the spirit of evil . . . When evil is suggested to you, when it arises in your hearts, it is through the temporal organization [the body]" (Young, 1925).

> 2 Nephi 2:30
> *I have spoken these few words unto you all, my sons, in the last days of my probation; and I have chosen the good part, according to the words of the prophet. And I have none other object save it be the everlasting welfare of your souls. Amen.*

Lehi's last statements in this chapter show his love for his children and his concern for their welfare. He says he has chosen "the good part." In other words, out of everything he could teach before he passes away, these doctrines are of the utmost importance. They are critical to our happiness and our salvation. As members of the Church, we are blessed to have access to these and the other essential truths that are found only in the Book of Mormon.

May we come to see the power of this book and how it can be a vital resource in our healing and recovery from childhood trauma. President Ezra Taft Benson said,

> *The Book of Mormon teaches us truth [and] bears testimony of Jesus Christ . . . But there is something more. There is a power in the book which will begin to flow into your lives the moment you begin a serious study of the book. You will find greater power to resist temptation. You will find the power to avoid deception. You will find the power to stay on the strait and narrow path. The scriptures are called "the words of life," and nowhere is that*

> *more true than it is of the Book of Mormon. . . . Every Latter-day Saint should make the study of this book a lifetime pursuit.* (Benson, 1986)

May we come away from reading these pages more aware of the necessity of the Atonement and how to access the blessings of this great sacrifice. May we come away with a greater understanding and gratitude for agency and opposition and the plan of salvation. May our minds be more aware of the adversary, his plan, and how to thwart him and his minions. May we be endowed with a greater desire to heal and to recover. And finally, may our hearts be filled with gratitude towards our Father in Heaven and our Savior Jesus Christ for their help and support and mercy and grace.

A SUMMARY OF CONCEPTS

When I read self-help books and spiritual-based books, I always underline passages and put stars next to specific paragraphs. Often I wish for a kind of "cheat sheet" at the end of the book that I could refer to—a list of highlights to refresh my memory. So I've done that here, pulling out some of the main points of advice and direction. Here, then, is a review of the basic concepts that will help you apply the Atonement to overcome childhood trauma:

- Remember that all unfairness will be made right by virtue of the Atonement.
- Maladaptive ways of handling trauma actually become the stumbling blocks that keep you from Heavenly Father and from accessing the Savior's Atonement.
- The brain is damaged by abuse and neglect, but it can also be healed. There is a physical component to healing from childhood trauma, as well as emotional and spiritual elements. In all areas of your life, you need the Atonement to help you heal.
- Hold fast—grab onto and cling to the iron rod (the word of God) when the going gets tough and when you feel hopeless or stuck.

- Work on understanding your relationship with and beliefs about God. The style of attachment you experienced as a child will directly impact the way you come to see yourself and the type of relationship you will have with God. Attachment styles are the template for current and future relationships, including your relationship with your Heavenly Family. These styles will impact how you relate to, connect with, and think about Heavenly Father, Jesus Christ, and the Holy Ghost. The more secure you feel in your relationships with your mortal, earthly parents, the more you will feel secure with Heavenly Father.
- Avoidant attachment: The spiritually avoidant person has, at his or her core, low self-esteem. Love has been experienced as conditional. If you have an avoidant attachment, you will routinely believe you are not good enough to be loved or validated. This idea must be attacked head on. Over and over and over, you must remind yourself that Heavenly Father loves you, regardless of your behavior. You must come to believe that your worth and value exists independently of your actions. Nothing you do can make you less than or more than in the eyes of God. Sometimes it may seem as though you need a sledgehammer to pound away at these twisted and distorted beliefs that are woven into your foundation.
- Anxious attachment: What someone with an anxious attachment needs to work on is faith—faith in God, faith in the concept of real love, and faith in themselves. If you have an anxious attachment, recognize and address your fear in every aspect of your relationships with others. You have been in a state of fear for so long that you may not always see the impact it is having in your life. Any and all distorted beliefs related to love need to be exhumed from

the buried foundation of your life. In this very elementary place of your personality will lie the artifacts that have tied love and fear together.

- Ambivalent attachment: Individuals who have an ambivalent attachment need to calm down, let go of control, and let God take over. If this is your attachment style, try to focus on developing faith and hope. Learn what a broken heart and a contrite spirit look and feel like. Stay out of other people's drama. Giving anonymous service is another good way to begin. Work constantly on positive self-talk. Study and understand the concepts of grace, justice, mercy, and Heavenly Father's love as they relate to the Atonement.
- Disorganized attachment: To overcome this attachment style and make a true, real connection to the Savior and His Atonement, a person must regain an internal connection with himself or herself. If this is your attachment style, you dissociate a great deal—disconnecting from emotions, internal sensations, and life experiences. Owning your life is paramount. You will need to reconnect, to plug back in to the physical and emotional network between the mind and heart, between the brain and body. Creating a safe environment is essential to help facilitate this reawakening. When you feel love, learn to sit with the experience and not run away from it. Over time, you will see God's love as safe and nurturing. This opens the door so you can experience the healing and restorative powers of the Atonement.
- Review faith and trust in God. Reconnecting to God is critical. Relearn who He is and what His personality is like. Throw away your outdated and false ideas about Him. This takes time, but the Holy Ghost will guide you

and give you the power to accomplish it. He will help you to see the incorrectness of some of your deeply held, perhaps even hidden beliefs about God. The Spirit will help you to discover the difference between your distorted beliefs and the actual truth. Once you divorce your abusers completely from who God is and how He feels about you, your faith can grow.

- Build belief in your worth and value. Faith is built on truth. And it is a lie that you are worthless and awful and no good. It is a lie that you are beyond God's help. It is a lie that Heavenly Father or Jesus or the Holy Ghost are unreliable and untrustworthy. It is a lie that your imperfections, character weaknesses, and sins make God love you less. It is also a lie that being perfectly obedient can somehow increase your worth and value. If these lies were true, you could make God love you or make Him hate you. Remember that you cannot change God's mind or create exceptions to rules and eternal laws.
- Faith requires truth. The truth is, regardless of what has happened to you or how the past has influenced your poor choices, God is the Father of your spirit and He loves you with an eternal and endless love. Nothing can ever change that.
- Learn to be open to emotions, especially love. Out of all the wide and varied emotions you can feel, love is undoubtedly the most healing, the most comforting, and the most nurturing. It is by far the most important emotion you, as an adult survivor of childhood abuse, can experience. There is no greater antidote to your loneliness than love. Not surprisingly, this emotion is also one of the most difficult to open up to and experience after having survived childhood trauma.

- Recognize reactions to fear. The key to overcoming trauma-based fear is awareness and becoming present. Become grounded in the here and now. Emotions are present oriented. The more you can be in tune with your emotions, the more you can stay in the moment, and the less likely you will be to overreact from a place of fear. We want to react from today, not from twenty or thirty years ago when we were scared children.
- Learning to know what you are feeling helps you become more aware of yourself. That awareness helps you to slowly but surely become comfortable in your body. (As a child, if you couldn't escape the person hitting you, yelling at you, or touching you, you could at least escape from yourself.) It is natural for you to stay disconnected from your body, even though you don't consciously do so. Feeling, connecting to, and expressing your emotions will connect you and bring you back into your body. It sounds very frightening, but this is the way to healing.
- Emotional awareness and trying to stay in the present moment are essential skills in accessing the Atonement of Jesus Christ. There is no healing by staying in the past. Healing can only happen in the present. The Atonement can only be accessed in the present moment of today.
- Pray for grace. Grace will help you connect to the Atonement. It helps to remove the aftereffects of abuse, both emotionally and physically. It will infuse strength beyond your own, enlighten your mind beyond your own comprehension, and soothe the painful muscle memory of past abuse. Grace will give your hope when you feel hopeless. It will helps rewire your brain, breaking apart old patterns that are outdated, twisted and distorted, and maladaptive. Grace will give you the

courage to feel emotions, to get back inside your body and feel alive again.

- What should the adult survivor of childhood trauma pray for? For grace—for spiritual abilities beyond your own to help you overcome the debilitating effects of the abuse you suffered. If you have been blinded by the past, pray for the spiritual gift of awareness and insight. If you have been hardened by the past, pray for a spiritually softened heart. If all you see is despair and darkness, pray for the spiritual gift of Christlike hope.
- The more you look for gratitude, the more the brain will focus on gratitude. Gratitude begets humility. Gratitude begets joy. Gratitude begets hope. Gratitude begets charity. Gratitude opens the door for you to feel and see the effects of grace in your life. You will begin to see more and more evidence of God's hands in your life. Whereas you once may have doubted that He even thought about you or cared about you, now with gratitude you will start to see His tender mercies on a daily basis.
- You are literally wired to directly access the Atonement. Your brain was made to connect to the effects of Christ's ultimate sacrifice. Your brain was made in such a way that as you try to live basic gospel doctrines, actual physical changes occur. The physical impact of past trauma in your brain can be reversed. Healing will happen. The principle of gratitude is just one example of how this occurs.
- The practice of mindfulness and empathy are among the most powerful agents of brain change known to science. Both acts strengthen the functioning of the prefrontal cortex to rewire old patterns. This means that when you see a situation clearly—when you are mindful or aware—and when you accept compassionately what you are

seeing (when you feel self-empathy), you can rewire old patterns without harming yourself. That is why God never counsels His children to hate themselves because of their sins or mistakes. Self-pity or self-hatred are not necessary requirements for change; in fact, they hinder change.

- Become willing to open yourself up to the enticings of the Holy Spirit. Open yourself to truth, to experience awareness, and to be able to connect the dots so you can make sense out of your present maladaptive reactions to the daily struggles of life. Breathe not from a shallow, ragged, fear-based place, but from your belly. Breathe deeply and fully, opening yourself physically and emotionally and spiritually. Follow the Spirit in becoming submissive—trusting God—willing to be humble and meek and patient.

Most of all, remember that the Atonement of Jesus Christ is real. It is meant for you to use in your daily life. It is the greatest tool of change given to humankind. Just as a laptop has ports for HCMI cables and USB cables that connect the computer to televisions, speakers, printers, external hard drives, etc., the same can be said for the human brain. You have "ports" where you can plug in spiritual "cables" from your brain to the Atonement. Those cables are made by and powered by the Holy Ghost. You can make the connections—plugging in the "cables"—through prayer, scripture study, grace, humility, gratitude, and forgiveness.

You are created, hard-wired, to connect to and utilize the power of the Atonement. That means every step you take in trying to find Christ and make your relationship with Him personal is facilitated by the biology of your body. Father in Heaven knew how hard this life would be for each of us. He knew we would be wounded—and that many of us would be wounded during the most vulnerable time period of our earthly sojourn. No matter what kind of evil the adversary has concocted for you, your Father in Heaven has already created an antidote and a way to heal you from the effects of that evil.

Trust your body. Trust God. Trust that the blueprint for change is already embedded in your mind and heart, only needing to be accessed. Trust that Jesus walks with you, feels your pain, your confusion, your anger, and your fear. Trust that He can truly understand what you are going through, and that you can feel supported by Him. Trust that you are not alone in those dark moments. Trust that if you reach out and try something different than what you've always done, there will be someone there to catch you, lift you, and prove that the new way works. This new way is Christ's way. I testify that His way works. I witness that His love cleanses us from the infected, black sludge of our abused past. I know that a rebirth is necessary and possible. I am not what my abuse told me I was. That person is gone. We can all be reborn through our Savior's great sacrifice. And if it can happen for me, I know it can happen for you. God loves you just as much as He loves me.

I know what I've written is true—that we can break free of the past and be made whole. I testify that the Atonement is powerful enough to find us, reach out to us, and bring us back into the loving embrace of our Heavenly Father and our Savior Jesus Christ. I owe Him everything, for He literally saved me. And like others who have been rescued by Jesus, I bear you my witness that hope is out there. Healing is real and available to all. It is available to you.

BIBLIOGRAPHY

Arehart-Treichel, Joan. 2001. "Evidence Is in: Psychotherapy Changes the Brain." *Psychiatric News*, 36(13) (July 6), 33.

Ballard, Melvin J. 1922. *The Three Degrees of Glory: A Discourse*. Salt Lake City, Utah: Deseret Book Co.

Benson, Ezra Taft. 1983. "What Manner of Men Ought We To Be." *Ensign*, Oct.

———1986. "The Power of the Word." *Ensign*, May.

Bradshaw, John. 1990. *Home Coming: Reclaiming and Championing Your Inner Child*. New York: Bantam Books.

Bremner, J. Douglas. 2000. "The invisible epidemic: post-traumatic stress disorder, memory and the brain." https://posttraumastressdisorder.wordpress.com/the-invisible-epidemic/.

Broderick, C. 2008. *The Uses of Adversity*. Salt Lake City, Utah: Deseret Book Co.

Cannon, George Q. 1894. *Millenial Star*. 23 Apr. 260.

ChildHelp. 2009. "Prevention and Treatment of Child Abuse." http://www.childhelp.org/pages/statistics.

Christensen, Byron R. 2013. Personal communication with author. October.

Christofferson, D. Todd. 2009. "Moral Agency." *Ensign*, June.

Clarke, Jean Illsley, Dawson, Connie. 1998. *Growing Up Again*. Center City, Minnesota: Hazelden.

Cochrane, H. 2003. "Adult attachment: best done early!" *YB-CP*, 1:3. Feb.

Cook, Quentin L. 2011. "Songs They Could Not Sing." *Ensign*, Nov.

Dapice, A., Inkanish, C., Martin, B., Brauchi, P. 2001. "Killing us slowly: when we can't fight and we can't run." www.dlncoalition.org/related_issues/killing_us_slowly.htm.

Dayton, Tian. 2000. *Trauma and Addiction: Ending the Cycle of Pain Through Emotional Literacy.* Deerfield Beach, Florida: HCI.

Dobberfuhl, Douglas. 2013. *Healing the Codependent Heart.* Salt Lake City, Utah: Walnut Springs Press.

Eyring, Henry B. 2010. "Trust in God, Then Go and Do." *Ensign,* Nov.

Faust, James E. 2007. "The Forces That Will Save Us." *Ensign,* Jan.

———2002. "The Lifeline of Prayer." *Ensign,* May.

———1979. "The Refiner's Fire." *Ensign,* May.

Finkelhor, D., Hotaling, G., Lewis, I. A., Smith, C. 1990. "Sexual Abuse in a National Survey of Adult Men and Women: Prevalence, Characteristics, and Risk Factors." *Child Abuse Negl.* 14(1):19–28.

Gerard, Jean M.; Buehler, Cheryl; Franck, Karen; Anderson, Owen. 2005. "In the Eyes of the Beholder: Cognitive Appraisals as Mediators of the Association Between Interparental Conflict and Youth Maladjustment." *Journal of Family Psychology,* vol. 19(3), 376–84.

Glass, Shirley. 2003. *Not "Just Friends": Rebuilding Trust and Recovering Your Sanity after Infidelity.* New York: Atria Books.

Goldberg, Susan. 2000. *Attachment and Development.* London: Arnold.

Goldstein, Jay A. 1996. *Betrayal by the Brain: The Neurological Basis of Chronic Fatigue Syndrome, Fibromyalgia Syndrome, and Related Neural Network.* Oxford, United Kingdom: Routledge.

Graham, Linda. 2013. *Bouncing Back.* Novato, California: New World Library.

Hafen, C. Bruce. 2008. *The Broken Heart.* Salt Lake City, Utah: Deseret Book Co.

———"The Value of the Veil." 1977. *Ensign,* June.

Hamilton, Kevin S. 2014. "Continually Holding Fast." *Ensign,* May.

Hinckley, Gordon B. 1994. "Save the Children." *Ensign,* Oct.

Holland, Jeffrey R. 2009. "Safety for the Soul," *Ensign,* Nov.

Hollander, E. et al. 2003. "Oxytocin Infusion Reduces Repetitive Behaviors in Adults with Sutistic and Asperger's Disorders." *Neuropsychopharmacology*. 28:193–98.

Hunter, Howard W. 1994. "Being a Righteous Husband and Father." *Ensign*, Oct.

Kikuchi, Yoshihiko. 2004. "Broken Windows, Broken Hearts," *Ensign*, Apr.

Kimball, Spencer W. 1978. "The True Way of Life and Salvation." *Ensign*, Apr.

Kolk, van der B. 1994. "The body Keeps the Score: Memory and the Evolving Psychobiology of Posttraumatic Stress. http://www.trauma-pages.com/vanderk4.htm.

Korb, Alex. 2012. "The neuroscience of giving thanks." *Pre-Frontal Nudity*. Nov.

McConkie, Bruce R. 1977. "The Salvation of Little Children," *Ensign*, Apr.

Monson, Thomas S. 1991. "Precious children—A Gift From God." *Ensign*, Oct.

National Sexual Violence Resource Center. 2012. Aug.

Oaks, Robert C. 2008. "Your Divine Heritage," *Ensign*, Apr.

Perry, B. 1999. Bonding and Attachment in Maltreated Children. *Child Trauma Academy*, 1 (4).

Pritt, Ann. 2001. "Healing the Spiritual Wounds of Sexual Abuse." *Ensign*, Apr.

Renlund, Dale G. 2015. "Latter Day Saints Keep on Trying." *Ensign*, May.

Scott, Richard G. 2008. "To Heal the Shattering Consequences of Abuse." *Ensign*, May.

———2007, "Using the Supernal Gift of Prayer," *Ensign*, May.

———2003. "The Sustaining Power of Faith in Times of Uncertainty and Testing." *Ensign*, May.

———2002. "To Be Free of Heavy Burdens." *Ensign*, Nov.

Steele, K., Van der Hart, O., Nijenhuis, E. 2001. "Dependency in the Treatment of Complex Posttraumatic Stress Disorder and Dissociative Disorders." *Journal of Trauma and Dissociation, 2 (4), 79–116.*

Stroufe, L. A., Duggal, S., Weinfield, N., Carlson, E. 2000. Ch. 5: "Relationships, Development, and Psychopathology." In Sameroff, A.J., Lewis, M., Miller, S. (eds.), *Handbook of Developmental Psychopathology* (2nd ed.). New York: Plenum Publishers.

Top, Brent L. 1988. *The Life Before: How Our Premortal existence Affects Our Mortal Life.* Salt Lake City, Utah: Bookcraft.

Turner, R., McGuiness, T. 1999. "Hormone Involved in Reproduction May Have Role in the Maintenance of Relationships." *Psychiatry,* July. http://www.oxytocin.org/oxytoc/.

Uchtdorf, Dieter F. 2006. "See the End from the Beginning." *Ensign,* May.

Walker, Joseph. 1992. "The Miracle of Change," *Ensign,* July.

Weber, Ellen. 2011. "A Brain on Forgiveness." *Practical Tactics from Neuro Discoveries.* Sept. 17.

Whitney, Orson F. 1918. "A Lesson from the Book of Job." *Improvement Era.* Nov.

Widtsoe, A. John. 1943. *Evidences and Reconciliations.* Collector's edition (1987). Salt Lake City, Utah: Bookcraft.

Wilcox, Brad. 2012. "His Grace Is Sufficient." *BYU Magazine,* Winter.

Wirthlin, Joseph B. 1993. "Spiritually Strong Homes and Families," *Ensign,* May.

Wolinski, Stephen. 1991. *Trances People Live.* Wilton Manors, Florida: Bramble Books.

Young, Brigham. John A. Widtsoe, ed. 1925. *Discourses of Brigham Young.* 1954 edition. Salt Lake City, Utah: Deseret Book Co.

Zohar, D., Marshall, I. 1999. *Spiritual Intelligence: The Ultimate Intelligence.* New York: Bloomsbury Publishing.

ABOUT THE AUTHOR

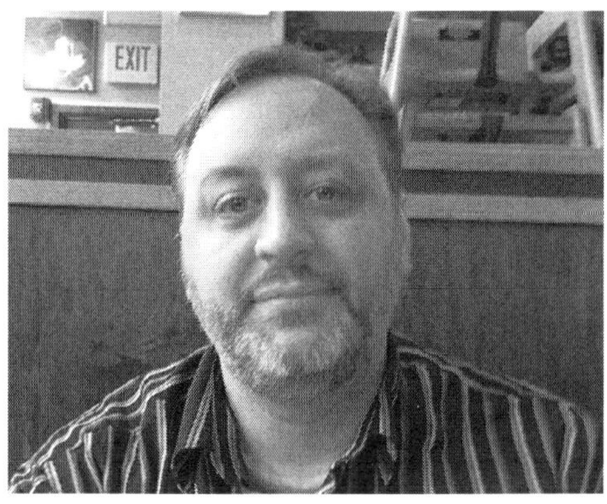

Douglas Dobberfuhl was born and raised in northwestern Wisconsin, where the snow was deep and the summers were humid. As a child, he could be found at the local swimming pool or immersed in a book. Doug served a full-time LDS Church mission in Brussels, Belgium. When he came home, he attended Brigham Young University. During his first semester at BYU, he met his future wife, Stephanie. She got his attention during a food fight at the Deseret Towers cafeteria. They were married six months later in the Los Angeles Temple and went on to have five children.

Doug received a masters of science degree in marriage and family therapy from Nova Southeastern University. He has worked as a counselor for twenty years. He has been a clinical supervisor, offered home-based counseling, done outpatient as well as inpatient work, and is the founder of The Center for Trauma and Addiction in Vancouver, Washington.

Doug also wrote *Overcoming Addiction: The Journey Begins*, *Overcoming Addiction: A Twelve-Step Companion Guide*, and *Healing the Codependent Heart.* He has been a contributing editor for

SheUnlimited online magazine, a woman's health and wellness periodical, as well as for A Second Opinion, a health and holistic-healing magazine. He is the author of *Using Scrapbooking to Heal from Childhood Trauma,* as well as many articles for treatment centers, including "Sexually Reactive Female Adolescents: Theory and Case Study," and "Intellectualizing: Denying Emotional States."

Please visit Doug's website, www.healingrecovery.org.

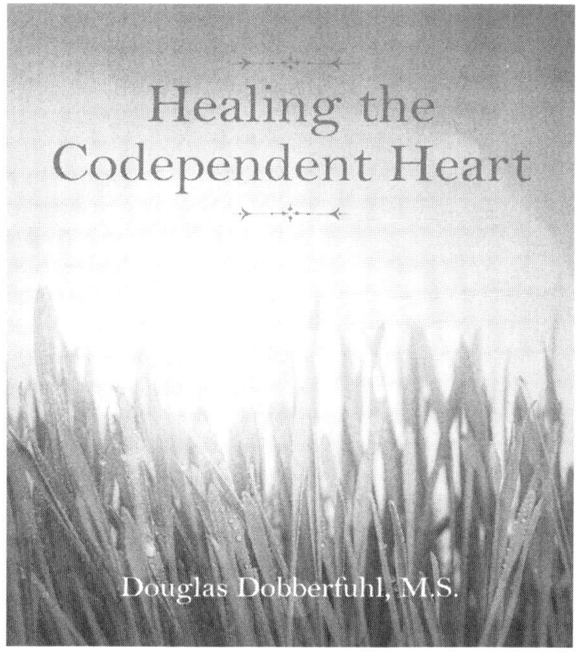

Do you struggle with seeing yourself as worthy and of value?
Does your happiness depend on others around you being happy?
Do you find yourself ruled by perfectionism?

When it comes to dealing with and overcoming the effects of this fallen, mortal world, there are essentially two paths to take. One encourages and supports us to manage our pain, hurts, and insecurities with willfulness and control. This path is called codependency. The other invites us to experience, learn, and become polished through our afflictions. This path is living in a state of charity. These two paths are often confused. Codependency can very easily look like and feel like charity. This book explores both subjects, drawing upon modern-day revelation, scriptures, and therapeutic experts in the field of codependency. Overcoming codependency is explored by teaching the reader how to apply the Atonement of Jesus Christ to this pervasive problem.

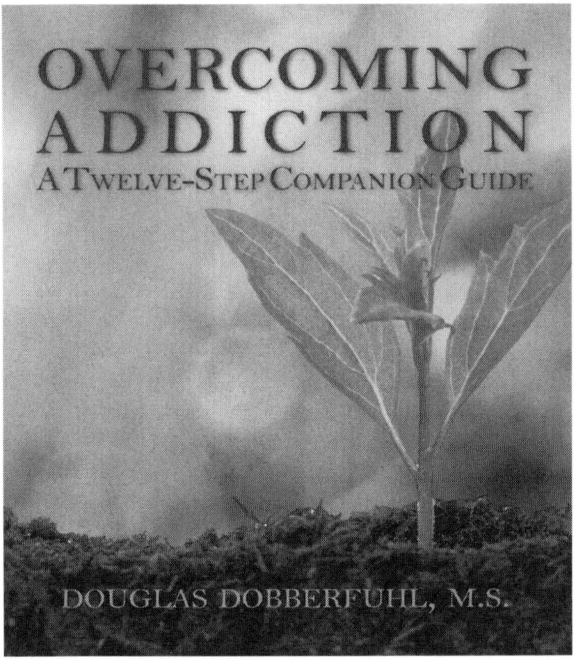

Overcoming Addiction: A Twelve-Step Companion Guide answers the often–asked question: "How do I work the Church's twelve steps?" With exercises, meditations, scriptural examples, and real-life stories of recovery, Overcoming Addiction is designed to be used hand in hand with the Church's addiction recovery manual. This companion guide helps the addict to more completely experience the power and promises of the twelve steps, and to apply the Savior's atonement to achieve lasting sobriety.

Overcoming Addiction is an essential tool for anyone struggling with addiction, as well as for family members of addicts and for professional counselors and addiction-recovery group leaders.